MOTIVATIONAL INTERVIEWING
IN HEALTH CARE

APPLICATIONS OF MOTIVATIONAL INTERVIEWING

Stephen Rollnick, William R. Miller, and Theresa B. Moyers, *Series Editors*

Since the publication of Miller and Rollnick's classic *Motivational Interviewing*, now in its third edition, MI has been widely adopted as a tool for facilitating change. This highly practical series includes general MI resources as well as books on specific clinical contexts, problems, and populations. Each volume presents powerful MI strategies that are grounded in research and illustrated with concrete, "how-to-do-it" examples.

MOTIVATIONAL INTERVIEWING in HEALTH CARE

Helping Patients Change Behavior

SECOND EDITION

Stephen Rollnick
William R. Miller
Christopher C. Butler

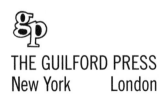

THE GUILFORD PRESS
New York   London

Library of Congress Cataloging-in-Publication Data

Names: Rollnick, Stephen, 1952– author. | Miller, William R. (William
   Richard), author. | Butler, Christopher, 1959– author.
Title: Motivational interviewing in health care : helping patients change
   behavior / Stephen Rollnick, William R. Miller, Christopher C. Butler.
Description: Second edition. | New York, NY : The Guilford Press, [2023] |
   Series: Applications of motivational interviewing | Includes
   bibliographical references and index.
Identifiers: LCCN 2022006804 | ISBN 9781462550371 (paperback) |
   ISBN 9781462550388 (hardcover)
Subjects: LCSH: Health counseling. | Motivational interviewing. | Health
   behavior. | Behavior modification.
Classification: LCC R727.4 .R65 2022 | DDC 610—dc23/eng/20220217
LC record available at *https://lccn.loc.gov/2022006804*

For practitioners on the frontline
—S. R.

For all who listen to their patients
—W. R. M.

To my best teachers,
the patients I have been privileged to serve
as a medical doctor
—C. C. B.

About the Authors

Stephen Rollnick, PhD, is Honorary Distinguished Professor in the School of Medicine at Cardiff University, Wales, United Kingdom. He is a cofounder of motivational interviewing, with a career in clinical psychology and academia that focused on how to improve conversations about change, and helped to create the Motivational Interviewing Network of Trainers (*www.motivationalinterviewing.org*). He has worked in diverse fields, with special interests in mental health and long-term health conditions like diabetes, heart disease, and HIV/AIDS. Dr. Rollnick has published widely in scientific journals and has written many books on helping people to change behavior. He is coauthor (with William R. Miller) of the classic work *Motivational Interviewing: Helping People Change*, now in its third edition. He has traveled worldwide to train practitioners in many settings and cultures, and now works as a trainer and consultant in health care and sports. His website is *www.stephenrollnick.com*.

William R. Miller, PhD, is Emeritus Distinguished Professor of Psychology and Psychiatry at the University of New Mexico. Fundamentally interested in the psychology of change, he is a cofounder of motivational interviewing and has focused particularly on developing and testing more effective treatments for people with alcohol and drug problems. Dr. Miller has published over 400 scientific articles and chapters and 60 books, including the groundbreaking work for professionals *Motivational Interviewing, Third Edition*. He is a recipient of the international Jellinek Memorial Award, two career achievement awards from the

American Psychological Association, and an Innovators in Combating Substance Abuse Award from the Robert Wood Johnson Foundation, among many other honors. The Institute for Scientific Information has listed him as one of the world's most highly cited researchers.

Christopher C. Butler, MD, is Professor of Primary Care at the Nuffield Department of Primary Care Health Sciences, University of Oxford, United Kingdom, and Professorial Fellow at Trinity College. He is Clinical Director of the University of Oxford Primary Care Clinical Trials Unit, and chairs the Longitude Prize Advisory Panel. Dr. Butler was for many years a general practitioner in South Wales. He was named the Wales Royal College of General Practitioners patient-nominated GP of the Year in 2019 and received the Royal College of General Practitioners Research Paper of the Year Award in 2020. His main research interests are in common infections, and health care communication and behavior change. He has led, or helped lead, over 30 clinical trials and published over 400 peer-reviewed papers.

Preface

This second edition of *Motivational Interviewing in Health Care* is written for frontline practitioners, whether you are a nurse, doctor, physical therapist, social worker, occupational therapist, dentist, diabetes educator, psychologist, behavioral health practitioner, or service manager. This book is about how to conduct skillful conversations that make a difference in people's lives, particularly when the focus is on why or how they might change. It has been completely rewritten by the cofounders of motivational interviewing (MI) and contains a new framework along with practical ideas, skills, and strategies for improving clinical practice.

Since the first edition of this text was published in 2007, the amount of research on MI has increased eightfold, including more than 1,700 clinical trials on a broad range of health topics. MI has been used to improve health behavior and lifestyle change outcomes against a background of a rise in long-term conditions like diabetes, heart disease, tuberculosis, and HIV/AIDS. Our grasp of how best to use MI in health care has been further tested and refined in clinical practice and practitioner training workshops. In this second edition, we use the simpler framework for MI offered in the third edition of the parent textbook, *Motivational Interviewing: Helping People Change* (Miller & Rollnick, 2013), in which we hope you will find accessible ways to tackle familiar challenges.

The well-being of practitioners is so often challenged by pressures of time and outcomes. In this updated edition, we give more attention to helping get the process right inside the consultation so that you feel less rushed and more effective. Making a transition from fixer to guide relieves you of the stress and weight of having to solve behavior change issues *for* patients, and instead help them to do this for themselves. In so doing, outcomes can also improve, along with your enjoyment of everyday practice.

What might you look for in this second edition? We address the merging of skillful advice giving with MI, helping you blend your professional expertise with evoking your patients' own wisdom and motivation. There are also new practical suggestions for offering not just praise but affirmation in everyday practice. There are chapters on how to merge assessment with MI, on very brief consultations, on how to run groups that are based on MI, and on how service managers can support the use of MI by making the front end of care more user-friendly.

At the heart of this book is clinical dialogue with commentary for getting the best out of scenarios that crop up every day, such as talking with a patient who feels reluctant to change, encouraging someone who lacks confidence, and raising the sensitive subject of change in the first place.

We are mindful, too, of the rewards and challenges of working on the frontline in marginalized communities, where patients face such daunting threats to their health and obstacles to change. There is hardly a medical condition in hospitals or community settings where the way people live their lives and the resources available to them do not directly impact their health and recovery. We hope this book will help you to feel more confident to work across boundaries of language and culture, because we pay careful attention to practical steps for engaging with people in an efficient manner, often under time constraints. The book contains numerous examples of practitioners speaking with people across cultures. The route to success is a very basic guideline: See this as a person first, patient second, and show them that you care. Then you can start developing your skills.

What's the best way to use this book? We suggest you dive into those parts that look the most helpful to you, with one proviso: Have a good read of the opening two chapters first, because they not only describe what MI is, but also highlight the all-important value of a fundamental shift in how you help patients to change. MI is a style of consulting, with an attitude behind it that will feel quite different from the "find it, fix it" approach that works well when managing acute medical presentations. The shift to working in this style starts inside you, where you hold back from solving problems for patients and adopt the mindset of a guide, focused on how to help people access their own strengths and abilities to achieve better health.

Consider some of these topics offered in the book:

- Get better at connecting with patients.
- Use advice giving more skilfully.
- Help the hesitant patient to resolve their ambivalence.
- Raise a difficult subject.
- Help patients to build their confidence and make change plans.
- Make your service environment more user-friendly.

We wish you well in developing and refining your style of practice and hope that above all you enjoy the perspectives presented in this book. From our own experience and that of others who have adopted MI into their professional practice, we are confident that if you step back from solving every problem for patients, your life becomes easier and your patients will become more empowered to make healthful decisions.

A note about language: In writing this book, we have made several decisions about language choices and style. For example, generally we refer to the people who come to us seeking treatment or medical care as "patients," though in places we may use "clients" or "people" instead. Furthermore, we have avoided as much as possible using technical or specialized terminology and jargon. Also, when a passage in the book calls for a pronoun referring to a singular, generic person, we use *they*, *them*, or *their* as that pronoun.

STEPHEN ROLLNICK
WILLIAM R. MILLER
CHRISTOPHER C. BUTLER

Acknowledgments

Members of the Motivational Interviewing Network of Trainers (MINT) have been hugely helpful in the writing of this book, offering new ideas and support in so many ways. As the book unfolded, its shape and content were influenced by conversations with these friends and with colleagues across the globe.

Our South African friends Goodman Sibeko, Loren Human, Fergus Ashburner, Zelra Malan, and Shaheema Allie have inspired us to look for ways of helping practitioners working under the strain of low-resource facilities in marginalized communities. Then there was this wonderful team who worked with us on vaccine hesitancy: Damara Gutnick, Alessandro Diana, Arnaud Gagneur, Patrick Bethiuame, Judith Carpenter, and Lynn Williams. We owe a special thanks to Nina Gobat for her work on agenda mapping and focusing. Nathan Wood, Pip Mason, Mike Porteous, Judith Carpenter, and Paul Warren gave generously of their time and fresh perspectives. Shaun Shelly, with his dedicated attention to what helpfulness involves, was an inspiration and more.

Finally, the staff at The Guilford Press was consistently kind and competent in helping us see the project through the writing and production process.

Contents

Prologue

All practitioners know the scenario where you invite a patient to change this or that behavior, and the response is one of ambivalence or even refusal. This dilemma is universal, as are efforts to persuade people out of the behavior. The problem is that simply telling others what to do is usually not enough to motivate them to do it. As we emerge from a pandemic, circling down on the health care practitioner is vaccine hesitancy, a good example of ambivalence if ever there was one. The subject of behavior change is not a fringe topic.

The genetics and biomarker revolutions in health care are beginning to deliver new and better targeted therapies. It's astounding how many presenting problems we considered untreatable only a decade ago are now managed well as part of a regular lifestyle, and even cured. With new technologies and new procedures, we are making great leaps in battling diseases. And yet all of these developments reinforce something we all know: The real breakthrough to better health and sustainable health care will involve individuals changing their own health-related behavior. Simply receiving magic bullet therapies will deliver very few of us from harm.

Of course, we don't need these newer medical technologies to identify what is making us sick and what will make us well. Smoking, excess alcohol, sedentary lifestyle, and poor diet account for most premature morbidity and mortality, and health care expenditure in developed countries. And communicable diseases are almost all influenced by human behaviors.

Indeed, is there a single illness, disease, or condition that will *not* be prevented or ameliorated by thinking or behaving differently? The

1

suffering caused by chronic pain, if we follow the evidence, can be greatly reduced by increasing activity, strength, and fitness. HIV can be prevented by condom use or postexposure prophylaxis (PEP), and largely controlled by adherence to daily medication; diabetes, cancer, and cardiovascular disease can be prevented or improved by weight loss, quitting smoking, exercise and healthy eating; influenza can be prevented by vaccination and hand washing; the most effective interventions for Huntington's disease and indeed dementia seem to be behavior change; unless those suffering with depression start to think and do things differently, the illnesses' tentacles will usually drag them back into its cruel grip.

Given the prevalence of health-related information, from clinicians, social media, and many other sources, it's clear that there are few people who engage in unhealthy behavior simply out of ignorance. Most unhealthy behavior brings both upsides and downsides for individuals. Smoking, for example, is one of the most toxic things you can do to your body; yet for many people, it remains a useful stress reliever, an exercise of autonomy and self-reward, an aid to weight loss, and one of the few ways they relax. In the 1970s, brief advice from general medical practitioners to their patients to quit smoking resulted in small, but important benefits at a population level. These days, however, there are few smokers who are ignorant of the health risks and of the medical profession's and society's disapproval of their habit. Those who persist in smoking don't lack information. They know the risks, and yet they enjoy the benefits. We have found that, no matter how entrenched the unhealthy behavior, its owner is, at some level at least, ambivalent about it.

Telling people what is good for them so often results in no change at best, and at worst, unhealthy behavior being even further entrenched. Knowing that, what do we do? How do *clinicians* rise to the challenge of helping people consider making changes appropriate to their health? How can practitioners minimize frustration at patients' persistence in things we know will harm them? Unless our clients and patients get into the driver's seat of their own behavior change challenges, progress will be limited and temporary. Can clinicians help unlock their patients' unique individual perspectives and creative energy to enable them to be their own physicians who then heal themselves?

CONSIDER: On the Frontline

Supporting outlying practitioners to engage with vulnerable people is a matter of life and death across vast swathes of Africa and other continents. Our interest in MI is in its adaptability and its direct relevance for engaging patients, otherwise vulnerable to dropout. Unfortunately, the inevitable intermingling of lifestyle behaviors in conditions like TB, HIV/AIDS and diabetes means that practitioners will burn out if all they do is hammer away at patients about this and that.

—GOODMAN SIBEKO, MD, PhD

Motivational interviewing (MI) offers a way this scenario can be navigated efficiently, with compassion and skill. It is not a panacea, and yet it can be incorporated into everyday practice to good effect.

PART I

INTRODUCTION TO MOTIVATIONAL INTERVIEWING

The essence of MI was clear to us from the outset 40 years ago: You get better outcomes if you put less pressure on patients to change, refrain from labeling or judging them, and instead help them to say why and how they might change, supported by offering your best advice when needed. Empathic listening is a powerful tool for helping them to do this.

In these opening two chapters, we lay the ground for the rest of the book, with the goal of describing the foundations on which MI rests (Chapter 1) and then what MI looks and feels like (Chapter 2). If some elements are familiar to you, we see this as a good sign that you will not need to completely reconstruct your usual consulting style but simply make adjustments to it. Small changes can have powerful impacts, like adjusting the footsteps of a dance or the grip position of a tennis racket.

One simple way of thinking about MI is to start with your mindset because this determines all else: You see your patients as people first, patients second, with strengths and wisdom that you can lean on and harness. You let go of what could be called a command style, a find-it-and-fix-it approach, to be replaced by a patient, calm, and altogether more satisfying way of approaching change for the patient—what we call a *guiding style* in Chapter 1. MI is rooted in this way of helping

people, and you will see this in the work of talented guides like teachers, sports coaches, and parents. No wonder then that MI will seem
familiar. The way these familiar ingredients are put together in MI
lends power, precision, and purpose to the conversation about change
that we hope you will enjoy getting better at. The way you speak to
people is as important as what you say to them.

CHAPTER 1

Good Practice

The Compassionate Guide

Good practice is an unsentimental commitment to doing good.
—AIDEN HALLIGAN

It was in the middle of a busy morning clinic, with a full waiting room outside, when she came in frankly reeking of alcohol, looking very unwell. I did a thorough physical examination, took blood, and asked her to come back a few days later for the results and a more thoughtful discussion. I never mentioned her drinking, apart from saying something like, "It's obviously pretty tough going for you at the moment." It simply felt unwise to raise the subject, especially given that my time had run seriously short. When she came back, I was expecting a difficult consultation because the blood result suggested a serious alcohol problem. I needn't have worried because she walked in and said, "Doctor I want to thank you. I stopped drinking. It was something you said last week." What had I said, I wondered? It emerged that I had apparently looked her straight in the eye as she left and said, "Don't be worried, I am going to see you through this over the next few weeks."
—CHRISTROPHER C. BUTLER

Conversations about change occur naturally throughout health care, planned and not, and conveying hope and kindness that sit at the heart of good practice takes no time at all. If people trust you, it makes a difference. In that example above, the practitioner's closing remark provides a signpost to what's involved: the *person* and the *relationship* is the primary focus, which makes it easier to address the patient *and* the problem.

Why do practitioners go into health care? Most report that they were motivated to do good, and that caring for others was a driving force for them from a young age. We expect that vision drove you into the field. Then, as you learned the craft of professional practice, it became necessary to build other skills into your portfolio, like detecting symptoms, making decisions about what intervention will help the most, and negotiating all sorts of things with patients. No question, in addition to practicing with compassion, you also need to be self-aware, nimble, knowledgeable, and socially skillful.

A common negotiating task arises when you want to provide guidance about why and how a patient might take action to improve their own health. How you conduct this conversation is important: You can't force a patient to change; only if *they* make a decision to change will they modify their behavior. This is what motivational interviewing (MI) is geared toward, and it also has other uses. For example, it can help you with:

- Assisting patients with challenges such as lifestyle change, vaccine uptake, and medication adherence.
- Helping them make up their own minds, free of pressure or coercion.
- Offering information and advice that patients appreciate, and act on.
- Forming strong relationships with them.
- Taking the heat out of conflict in the consultation.
- Listening well without losing control of time.
- Making plans for action that patients take ownership of.

The aim of this book is to build on your existing skills, to improve your self-awareness of how you develop trust and relationships that make a difference, and to improve outcomes for patients in the interest of their health and well-being.

Conversations about Change

Have a look at this exchange, which is most definitely not MI, but rather the kind of conversation that gave rise to it:

PRACTITIONER: Okay, so it's time to ask you to take a vaccination for COVID. It's really important that we give this to every patient these days.

PATIENT: Yes, I know you want this, but I don't think it's a good idea because it's all too much of a rush and because the politicians want us to. Why should we trust them?

PRACTITIONER: As a doctor, I can tell you that taking this vaccine will help others, too, to cut down the rate of infection in this very community.

PATIENT: I'm not sure I believe that anyway; I heard that those medicine companies are just doing this for their fat profits, and who knows how it might harm us in this community. It's happened before, so why can't it happen again?

PRACTITIONER: I can only tell you that many people are dying of this virus right now. Can you see that?

PATIENT: Yeah, sure, like they do every year with flu.

We are not suggesting you practice like this, but you might nevertheless recognize the pattern. Correcting and persuading people to change can be problematic, and this is probably why MI has such potential to be helpful in health care.

It is no secret that when you stop trying to oblige people to change, they seem more open to the idea, a lesson we authors learned through many conversations in a health care situation. We learned another lesson, too: how *efficient* it can be to listen to patients. Our experiences working with patients changed us as people and practitioners, and learning MI allowed us to build on what we did every day. Other everyday tasks became more satisfying all around.

> **When you stop trying to oblige people to change they become more open to changing.**

Returning to the exchange above, how likely is it that this patient will move toward getting a vaccination? Not very, right? An effort that started from a genuine desire to help the patient ends up in a discouraging battle of wills. If the next three consultations follow a similar arc, the clinician may well start to feel downhearted, if not depleted. And, the patients may well leave the clinic frustrated and feeling they have not been heard or understood, certainly not uplifted about improving their health.

The above exchange was driven by a desire to be helpful and took the form of an effort to solve the patient's problems *for* them, which is something patients expect and appreciate with many presenting medical complaints. And yet, ironically, providing (or prescribing) solutions is not a particularly helpful approach when what needs to change is someone's behavior. What's usually behind a prescriptive approach is something we refer to as the "righting reflex"—the almost unconscious inclination to fix things and set them right, a well-ingrained habit that can be traced back to that desire to do the best for people.

Good practice is surely more than repeating messages about how to get healthy. How can you get those messages to stick? Or, more precisely, how can you use your time with patients such that they get the most out of their visit? What we aspire to offer you in this book is a way of tweaking the conversations you have about change, where your best advice can be embraced and your timely interventions be actively joined by a patient who feels hopeful and empowered.

> **How can you use your time so patients get the most out of their visit?**

What Do Patients Want?

Most patients who come to a clinic or other health care service want to be treated and respected as capable individuals. They also want to trust, to be heard—and understood—whether they are feeling anxious, confused, hopeful, or even pessimistic at the prospect of another consultation.

What can you do to meet those wishes, particularly when you know a patient might need to make an adjustment in diet, be more consistent taking medication, drink less alcohol, receive a vaccine, or be more active? What does good practice involve here? Many patients will appreciate your best advice if they feel you are trustworthy and care about them. However, they are also likely to vary in their motivation to change. Some will readily want to know the facts and to understand why they should change, some will waver and hesitate to commit, and others will want to rebuff your efforts or even run away as fast as they can.

One thing patients will probably all appreciate is freedom of choice, room to decide for themselves why and how they might change their lives. If they feel this freedom is being threatened, it is only human for them to react against your advice, as the patient in the exchange above seemed to do. What seemed straightforward to the practitioner felt like a challenge to the patient. They seemed to know quite a lot already about what will and will not be achievable in their life, and the conversation served at best to reinforce their assumptions.

How Can You Help?

How might that earlier conversation about getting a vaccine have gone differently? Your best work surely goes beyond spotting what needs to happen and then telling patients what to do. It calls for connecting with them and showing you appreciate what it's like from their side. And, it involves using their own knowledge and wisdom about how they might make changes that can lead to better health and well-being. Helping people to change involves more than simply fixing things that are wrong with them. It involves recognizing their agency and then giving them tools to do the fixing themselves. But under the crush of caseloads, how do you keep this in mind, bring your best game so that your patients step up to be part of the treatment team? From your side, this will involve both compassion and skill.

The Style of a Guide

One way to get the most out of patient conversations about change is to consider a shift in style, from being a director to being a *guide*. This style forms the foundation of MI, where your role is to draw out from patients why and how they might change, where you start with the wisdom and abilities of the person in front of you, much like a travel or mountain guide might, ready to provide advice and information here and there as needed.

Consider this style in relation to two others: a directing style and a following style. Each has its own time and place (see the box below), and in any conversation the idea is to pick the style that best matches the present circumstances.

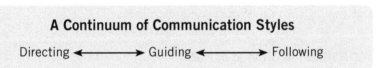

A Continuum of Communication Styles

Directing ⟷ Guiding ⟷ Following

You can sharpen your judgment about when to switch styles and sharpen your skills within each style. For example, if you want to get better at giving advice, you might focus on how a directing style can be used more skillfully. You can use the skills of MI to do this, seamlessly merging helpful advice giving with MI. If, however, your priority is to get better at listening, what will it mean to use a following style more skillfully, for example, if a patient walks in clearly tearful and in need of being heard?

Somewhere between directing and following is the guiding style mentioned above. Guiding is the focus of this book, or as one practitioner put it, "I like to stand with my two feet firmly in the guiding style and move to either side as needed." This style is recognizable in everyday life, used by people like parents, teachers, and sports coaches when they want to encourage someone to learn, adapt, or make their own decisions about what to do. With MI being merely a refinement of this style, it's no wonder that practitioners hear about MI and remark, "I do a lot of this stuff quite naturally." Indeed, it is a style you may already know about, and the case for sharpening its use seems well justified.

Using a guiding style harnesses some powerful drivers of learning and change in those you treat. For example:

- You view them as people first, patients second.
- You place high value on connecting well.
- You work with their strengths, not only their problems or deficits.
- You champion choice and believe your patients are capable of making wise decisions about their lives.
- You *offer* advice rather than impose it.

If you find yourself nodding in agreement with these principles, then guiding may serve you well as a consulting style. The inspiration for many practitioners lies in breaking away from being the "deficit detective," who is on the hunt for things that are wrong with the patient. Having that mindset is useful when diagnosing, but dysfunctional when empowering someone. Instead, while you might need to assess, diagnose, and suggest solutions to problems, with the guiding style your vision is a broader one, where you place high value on engagement, empowerment, and making the best of the patient's strengths.

CONSIDER: A Change of Heart

People come to my clinic with little hope of improving their health, weighed down by social stress, poverty, and all kinds of problems. I used to feel that I had to always tell them what was right and what to do, like I was a good health policeman. My mental health suffered because I could see also that they found it hard to listen, let alone act on my suggestions. The idea of me being their guide rather than the "health instructor" was a big shift for me. I have my bits of advice, but I now start somewhere different, by engaging with them, and then we are able to work together. That's when I try to be the compassionate guide, offering advice but always trusting what they think also.

—Nozipho Majola, *Lifeline Durban Gender-Based Violence Programme, South Africa*

Making Every Conversation Count

Everyone has their own attitude toward patient care, ways of handling consultations, decision trees, and favorite questions, and no doubt you refine these as the years go by. Sometimes these aids work well, other times less so. Roadblocks to progress in a clinical conversation can appear regularly, like when you feel unable to get through to a patient, hesitant about raising a difficult subject, or baffled by what you believe is an obstacle created by the patient themself. How might you make even small adjustments to your routines to keep such roadblocks to a minimum?

We designed the scenarios that follow here to highlight familiar challenges and to consider some routes to good practice. You will notice places we point to in later chapters where you can dig a little deeper into topics of interest to you.

The Scenario: Engaging and offering information.

The Challenge: A patient is offered a vaccination and says it will do him more harm than good. A tiring battle of wills could flare up if you raise the subject abruptly and then hammer away at the patient, trying to convince him that your view is the best one. The clues lie in your language and the patient's defensive reaction:

> CLINICIAN: *I need to tell you* that failure to have this vaccination could result in . . .
>
> PATIENT: Yes, but I don't believe this because . . .

Good Practice: How do you connect well and efficiently, and offer advice that allows the patient to make a well-informed choice? If you engage well, using core skills like open questions and listening statements, however briefly (see Chapter 7), it will be much easier to raise the need for the vaccine, using language that is nonthreatening: "May I ask your permission to raise the subject of this vaccination for . . . ?" Then you can offer, not impose, information and advice (see Chapters 11 and 17). Few patients are 100% against a vaccination. A sizable number are in favor, and many are wavering, hesitant, or what we call ambivalent. A few minutes spent offering information and championing their choice will reap rewards.

The Scenario: Finding the focus for lifestyle change.

The Challenge: With long-term chronic conditions, in any setting, how people conduct their lives will affect their condition. Add poverty and mental health issues to the mix, where life can feel like a matter of "just getting by," and the conversation about change is potentially complex. Many will have "heard it all before"—about the need to change lifestyle behaviors—and they could be sensitive to feeling blamed for their medical condition. Assuming you engage with the person, how do you then make a decision about whether to focus on one change target (e.g., diet) and not another (e.g., exercise)? How does the patient see your role here, and how much guidance do they want?

Good Practice: Can this be a shared decision? How does this negotiation unfold? To begin with, people will appreciate you asking about their lives with an open mind. Then you will want to make a decision *with* them about which direction to go in, what kind of change is going to be most useful to focus on first, and why. Coming to these decisions requires transparency on your part and tuning into what makes sense to them in such a way that they feel involved and empowered to make changes, and are open to your ideas, too. Additionally, you don't want to be overly directive; neither do you want to stand back passively, not giving the patient any indication of what you think. This focusing process involves a skillful negotiation, and sometimes you will need to put your own views to one side in favor of following those of the patient (see Chapter 8).

The Scenario: Evoking motivation for change.

The Challenge: Nearly every day you find yourself recognizing there's a single, specific change that is in a patient's best interests to make—for example, using a hearing aid, stopping smoking, taking a new medication, or losing weight. You raise the subject with good intention, then you get a "Yes, but . . ." reply, a blank look, or a quiet nodding of the head. Have you jumped too far ahead of the patient's readiness? Have you fallen into that persuasion trap, where the harder you press your point, the more you get pushback?

Good Practice: If you have only a couple of minutes, how can you make the best use of time to help the patient resolve their doubt or uncertainty? Here's where shifting to a guiding style might be useful, with a few open questions that give the patient a moment to say why and how they might change, and some time for you to offer advice, should they want it. The skills involved in drawing out the wisdom of the patient are described in Part II, and this kind of conversation is what MI was designed for (see Chapter 9). Only the patient can change their behavior!

The Scenario: Planning for change.

The Challenge: Consider a consultation with a smoker, who knows all the facts, wants to quit, but feels weighed down by stress and everyday life and simply doesn't believe they can go without cigarettes. Lack of confidence is a common obstacle to behavior change. What might seem clear enough to you feels more difficult for the patient. If you tell them what to do, the suggestion often fails to change behavior.

Good Practice: How ready is the patient to do something? Is it *just* a lack of confidence, is the timing not right, or are they not truly convinced about the benefits of change in the first place? Rather than assuming you have to work out all of this, you can just ask them. A skilled guide will empathize with how the patient is feeling, and also conversationally come alongside as they search for a solution together, without you applying pressure. A few moments spent pausing to reflect *together* on the patient's ambivalence, and to consider what has helped others, can reap rewards. Planning well is best driven by skillful conversation, with a keen eye on the strengths of the patient (see Chapter 10).

A set of common communication challenges run through scenarios like those above: connecting well (engaging), agreeing what change to make (focusing), building motivation (evoking), and making change plans that are realistic and promote the confidence to succeed (planning). These tasks mirror the framework for MI presented in the next chapter and the key chapters in Part III.

Looking After Yourself

Practitioner well-being is one of the most important drivers of good practice, and this can be undermined by feeling that you have to solve every problem that comes your way. This is a commonly reported experience among health care practitioners, and it contributes to compassion fatigue, burnout, and suboptimal care, particularly in low-resource settings with high patient turnover. A shift to using a guiding style and MI can have a noticeable positive effect on practitioner well-being. You step away from viewing a patient list as a set of tasks to be carried out *on* people, where you find yourself going through the same routines and repeating the same messages time and again. Every patient is a unique person, and your role is to support, inform, and encourage them to find their best route to better health.

> **CONSIDER: What Gets You Up in the Morning?**
>
> I went into health care because I wanted to help people because I care about them. At some point I got burned out and it was harder for me to connect with my patients. Learning about MI gave me the tools to connect with them in a way that was effective, time-efficient, that got me the outcomes—and it brought joy back into my work.
>
> —Damara Gutnick, MD

MI draws its inspiration from the attitude of a committed and caring guide. The responsibility for change is viewed as a shared one; the consultation is free of pressure and disagreement because in the end it is the patient's choice whether to change or not. Seen in this light, good practice in health care involves not just looking after patients but looking after yourself, too.

Good practice means not just looking after patients but looking after yourself.

When the Conversation Begins

This chapter has focused on a broad perspective on good practice, which serves as the foundation for MI. We now turn to what MI is, why it helps, and what it looks like. One of the most common challenges is patient ambivalence about change, when you hear mixed messages like "I know I am overweight . . . but what else can I do?" or "I'll see what I can do. I hardly get time to sleep these days." What could you say that will be helpful? If persuading them won't help, what will? We submit, this is where MI comes into its own. Our experience has been that the MI approach can be used in many corners of health care, including in quite tough circumstances.

Conclusion

MI is a style and set of skills for tackling diverse challenges. It is not the right tool for every patient and every problem, but nevertheless it is capable of being integrated into everyday practice. For example, you can use MI to improve the way you offer information and advice. It essentially involves anchoring you in a guiding style to get the best out of your patients, helping them to say what they want and need. MI can help in brief exchanges or in longer sequences of conversation; as a stand-alone intervention or merged with other tasks; and used by practitioners of all kinds, both newcomers and seasoned professionals.

This book will take you through what MI is (Part I) and the core skills you use to navigate consultations efficiently and effectively (Part II). We then provide practical examples of how you can use and refine the way you connect with patients, establish a focus for change, draw out their best motives for changing, and make plans for change that stick (Part III). Finally, we turn to everyday challenges, such as offering advice, working remotely or in groups, brief conversations, and how to integrate MI with assessment (Part IV).

In essence, this book is a call to highlight and refine the skills you already have; to bear in mind the attitudes of compassion, curiosity, and respect that underlie MI; and to then adapt MI to your needs.

CHAPTER 2

Motivational Interviewing

People are generally better persuaded by the reasons which they have themselves discovered than by those which have come into the mind of others.

—BLAISE PASCAL

In 2006 I ran this MI training workshop on a pediatric ward of a large teaching hospital in Cape Town, South Africa. It was during the height of the HIV/AIDS pandemic and newly acquired antiretroviral therapy offered the promise of saving the lives of babies, and their mothers. Adherence was therefore the focus of the workshop. It was a difficult assignment because not only was I was working across barriers of language and culture, but the participants were themselves mothers, volunteer counselors, many of whom were unwell and infected with the virus. A year later I returned for a follow-up visit, and a mother came up to me and said, "That workshop was really helpful. I went home and decided to stop trying to make my son change his ways. Instead, I used that guiding style and we have been getting on so much better. He knows that I care, and we have much better conversations about how he wants to get on in life."

—STEPHEN ROLLNICK

The guiding style described in the last chapter formed the foundation for the workshop described above, and this mother made full use of it and some insights from MI to shift her attitude and behavior with her son at home. She put less pressure on him to change, and switched her approach from "I know what's best for you" to "Here's what you might do, what do you think?"

In taking on the style of a guide, you invite the patient to be in the driver's seat, supported by you alongside. This can seem both comfortingly familiar and a challenge to integrate. Yet with a little patience and practice, you can soon reap the rewards. This involves awareness of how best to unleash patient motivation and how to avoid a few common pit-falls, too.

What Is MI?

MI is a form of patient-centered care, a particular way of having a con-versation about change in which you seek to strengthen patients' own motivation for and commitment to do what is needed. The task involves a sometimes radical shift in mindset for many practitioners—you help them say why and how they might improve their health, not solve this question for them. The starting point is to view them as people first, patients second.

The Spirit of MI

When patients walk into the room, can they tell what your attitude toward them is? No doubt, your greeting and friendly manner will help, and we suggest you expand on that manner with what we call the "spirit of MI." This spirit, fundamental to MI, is a combination of *working well in tandem* and *facing forward toward change*, toward an improve-ment in patient health and well-being. It is like you are walking along-side your patient, not in circles, but down a path toward change. You are the guide, and the ideal is, once you have both agreed on what path to walk down, the patient walks freely toward change as far as they feel is right. To stretch the metaphor a little, if you and the patient walk off the path into brambles or wander down into a cul-de-sac, your job is to help get back on track.

There are four elements of this MI spirit.

Partnership

Because you can't fix other people's behavior, change requires a side-by-side collaboration between your professional expertise and their life experience. People appreciate, need, and take strength from a helpful relationship. We highlight the skills involved throughout this book.

Acceptance

An empathic, nonjudgmental attitude helps make MI work: accepting patients as they are, and recognizing their irrevocable right

> **When patients feel accepted as they are, they are more able to change.**

to choose how they will live their lives. Ironically, when patients experience being accepted as they are, they are more able to change. Respectful listening to patients' own perspectives is a powerful way to convey acceptance. You show respect for, and work with, people's own wisdom and resources.

Compassion

What we mean by compassion is a Hippocratic commitment to alleviate suffering, do no harm, and promote patients' health and well-being. MI is not a way of getting people to do what you want them to do or what is in your own interest. Rather, it is a way of helping them make changes that they perceive as important within their own values and goals.

Empowerment

MI is about calling forth that which patients already have within them: their own values, ideas, caring, and motivations to change. To combine your best advice with the wisdom of the patient is what we mean by empowering. It involves practicing as a skillful guide. MI honors patients' autonomy and ability to change. You cannot make life changes for them, so you empower them to do it themselves. *What* health-related changes would this patient be willing and able to make? *Why* might they be willing to do it? *How* could this change best be accomplished and fit into the patient's life? All of these are topics not for prescription, but for negotiation. No one knows more about your patients than they do, and you need their collaboration if changes in behavior and lifestyle are to occur.

Partnership, Acceptance, Compassion, and Empowerment. These four perspectives on practice—PACE yourself—describe a state of mind and heart within which MI is best practiced. Without this perspective, there is a danger of using skills "on" patients, rather than with them. When MI is done well, you are helping patients literally talk themselves into change. Any advice or information you have is best offered to support their own good reasons to change. When done well, it feels like a very normal and recognizable conversation. Also, note that MI is not just about being warm and friendly, not just about being patient-centered, but also about being patient-centered, but also involves you facing in the direction of healthy changes, purposefully pointing the conversation toward how they might come about.

MI is not just about being warm and friendly, but involves facing in the direction of healthy change.

Four Processes of MI

If a consultation is like a journey, what might this journey look and feel like if you are using MI? What will you do to empower the patient to change? We developed a four-processes model to help practitioners make better progress. These processes are Engaging, Focusing, Evoking, and Planning. They are not linear steps or stages, but rather four activities that occur within MI. The skills of Asking, Listening, Affirming, and Summarizing (described in more detail in Part II) are useful in all four processes. The first of them, engaging, involves developing and maintaining a supportive, trusting provider–patient relationship. The remaining three processes are all geared toward helping the patient to clarify what they might do to achieve better health, and why and how they might do it.

Engaging

The metaphoric question in engaging is "Can we take a walk together?" Whatever the concerns patients may bring through the door with them, they have a story to tell. Engaging is about listening well to that story, and keeping a good connection throughout the consultation. It doesn't have to take a lot of time. It's more about giving patients your full and curious attention. Little change is likely to happen without a solid foundation of engaged provider–patient relationship.

Focusing

The next metaphoric question on the journey of MI is "Where are we going?" This is actually the *what* question: What kind(s) of change would your patient be willing to discuss and consider in the interest of health? There are, for example, quite a few ways in which patients with diabetes can change their behavior and lifestyle for longer-term quality of life. Providing a list of recommended changes is unlikely to have much impact. What one or two changes might this patient be interested in talking about on this visit? Choosing where to start is a negotiation process. Beginning in Chapter 4, we offer some practical skills for focusing well during your dialogue.

Evoking

Once you have a change goal or focus for discussion, a central task on the MI journey is to consider together *why* your patient might choose to make this change. You do have, from your professional expertise, good ideas about what health-relevant changes to recommend, and why it would be a wise idea to make those changes. A temptation is simply to *tell* patients why they should do it, but the evoking process involves dis-covering each patient's *own* motivations for positive health change. What is more likely to activate patients is for them to freely choose what changes to make and express their own motivations for doing so. The metaphoric question at this point is "Why do you want to go there?" A broad question in consultation, for example, is "What do you need your health for?" (Rakel, 2018). It is important that patients make the argu-ments for change, that they literally voice reasons and desires that would make the effort of change worthwhile. We will come back to this shortly when discussing "change talk."

> **It is important that patients make the arguments for change.**

Planning

A fourth metaphoric question on the MI journey is "How will you get there?" After negotiating *what* change to consider and *why* the patient would be willing to make it, comes consideration of *how* best to accom-plish it. Again, there is the temptation just to tell patients how to do it, but planning is a negotiation process, evoking the patient's own ideas and preferences. Even with something as concrete as compliance in taking medication, there are many ways to do it right. Where will the medication be kept? How will prescribed dosing fit into this person's daily routine? What might be good reminders? Could someone else help the patient with medication. What if a dose is missed? To address such issues, you need the patient's cooperation and their own knowledge.

Ambivalence

These consultations about change are like a dance that can unfold smoothly, proceed with a few bumps and stumbles along the way, and even go horribly wrong at times. Ambivalence about change rears its head often and requires thoughtful handling.

CONSIDER: The Dance of Ambivalence

When we first developed MI, back in the 1980s, we noticed how placing pressure on people to change had a negative effect on the atmosphere in the conversation and on their willingness or motivation to change. The major shift for us was to hold back from labeling or blaming the patient and instead to practice acceptance and give them space to breathe and explain what might motivate them to change. Then we noticed the phenomenon of ambivalence, a conflict for them about whether to change or not. How we responded here could trip up the dance or lift the conversation to new heights that helped people break free from the grip of this uncertainty about change. We never tried to develop a theory of MI, but over the decades we have repeatedly highlighted this single word of ambivalence like a signpost that cannot be ignored.

—WILLIAM R. MILLER AND STEPHEN ROLLNICK

With the benefit of hindsight and many stumbles through consultations ourselves, we can now clarify a few fundamentals for navigating how best to approach a patient who is feeling ambivalent about change. They might want to change, and can see the benefits of doing this, *and* at the same time they can also feel a pull toward not changing. The challenge for both parties is to avoid a conflict of wills in which you, the practitioner, argue in favor of change and the patient reacts against this and gives voice to why change is not a good idea. "Why don't you consider doing . . . " is all too often met with "Yes, but you see I don't think that will work because. . . ." To put it simply, change happens when people *themselves* perceive and accept good reasons to do so, a truth captured well by 17th-century philosopher Blaise Pascal in the opening quote for this chapter. When using MI, you invite the patient to express their ambivalence, acknowledge both sides of the dilemma, and focus particularly on the positive, the case for change. How you do this is illustrated in many places in this book. In this introductory chapter on MI, here are some fundamentals we have identified, based on what we have learned about how people change successfully:

- Ambivalence is a normal human experience.
- Avoid solving the conflict for them or pressuring them to change.
- Demonstrate acceptance of them and the dilemma they face. This goes a long way to helping them feel safe enough to break free of it, as does championing their freedom of choice.
- Ask them how they see things, and particularly about why and how healthy change might come about. Use listening skills to reflect back their own good motivations to change.
- If a patient remains uncertain, or decides not to change, that is not a bad outcome. Change often occurs at a later point in time.
- Some patients might want information or advice. Ask them, and

if they do want it, offer this as a trusted and compassionate messenger.

These are some guiding principles for the evoking process described earlier in the chapter. For the practitioner, evoking usually feels like you are getting out of the patient's way while they say why and how they might change. For the patient, it can be the first time anyone has given them the space to breathe and to think aloud about how to break free of ambivalence. This thinking often leads gently to the question of how they might lift their confidence to make changes, which is where the planning process comes to the fore.

Offer information or advice as a trusted and compassionate messenger.

The Language of Change

When talking with patients about change, it makes good intuitive sense to pay attention to the language they use because this language is an expression of their motivation to change. "I maybe should . . ." is quite different from "I am definitely going to. . . ." MI at its simple and elegant best involves encouraging people to express their motivation to change, calling for this language, and then reflecting it back to them, like holding a mirror for them to notice and explore further.

When people express aloud in another's presence the intention to take action and a plan for doing it, they are more likely to take that action (Gollwitzer, 1999). The more people voice arguments for rather than against change, the more likely it is to happen (Magill et al., 2018, 2019). It is ideal, then, to arrange consultations so that patients voice their own motivations for healthful change. If you tell patients what, why, and how they should change, the predictable response is "Yes, but . . . ," which is just the opposite of voicing motivations for change. This is perfectly normal and expected when someone is ambivalent, as most people are when faced with making a change.

Change Talk and Sustain Talk

"Change talk" is the language people use that moves them in the direction of making a change. If you listen carefully to what your patients say, you will notice this kind of speech, and it matters. Decades of research have clarified some specific types of change talk that are often heard in conversation (see the Appendix on the research of MI at the end of the book). Some types of change talk signal that a person is considering or leaning toward change. For example:

- Desire: "I *want* to stay healthy."
- Ability: "I think I *could* do that."
- Reasons: "My blood pressure is getting too high."
- Need: "I've *got to* lose some weight."

Other kinds of change talk indicate that a patient is deciding or preparing to make a change:

- Willingness: "I would be willing to take a walk most days."
- Commitment: "I am *going to* do this now."
- Taking Steps: "I have already talked to my daughter about walking with me."

An early step in developing skillfulness in MI is attuning your ear to recognize change talk, so you know that when you hear patients say these things, you have heard something important.

"Sustain talk" is the flip side of change talk: things people say that move them away from making a change. Very similar kinds of speech can move patients toward (change talk) or away (sustain talk) from making a change. Table 2.1 lists some things a patient might say to you about

TABLE 2.1. Smoking Cessation: Change Talk versus Sustain Talk

	Change talk	Sustain talk
Desire	"I *wish* I could quit."	"I really *enjoy* smoking."
Ability	"I *could* probably do it."	"I don't think I'm *able* to quit."
Reasons	"My kids would be happy if I did."	"Smoking is the only way I can relax."
Need	"I've really *got to* quit."	"I don't think I *have to* quit."
Willingness	"I'm *thinking about* quitting."	"I'm not *ready* to quit."
Commitment	"I'm going to quit."	"I will keep on smoking."
Taking Steps	"I got rid of all my ashtrays today."	"I bought three cartons today."

quitting smoking, divided into those statements that represent change talk and those that represent sustain talk.

See how it works? People essentially argue for or against making a change, and often both. It is quite common, especially when someone is feeling ambivalent, to hear both change talk and sustain talk in the same utterance; for example, "Yeah, I could I suppose, but then how will I cope when I feel stressed?" or "I can see why you think I should lose weight, but you should see the food we eat. We can't afford all those expensive healthy foods." The word "but" often separates change talk from sustain talk.

The Patient Tips the Balance

Although you may not have thought about these particular subtleties of language, you already know it's worth paying attention to what people say. For example, when you ask a person to do something, you listen carefully to what they say in response because the words contain important clues as to whether it's going to happen. The more change talk and the less sustain talk you hear, the greater the likelihood that the person will do it. It's just part of normal social discourse.

What we now know from MI research is that the ratio of a person's change talk to sustain talk predicts change, and is very much a product of social interaction (Glynn & Moyers, 2010; Magill et al., 2018, 2019; Moyers & Martin 2006). What *you* say and how you say it during consultations influence your patients' balance of change talk and sustain talk. You can speak in a way that evokes patients' arguments for or against change, and it matters. The more your patients verbalize their own desire, ability, reasons, and need for change, the more likely it is to happen. Conversely, if you mostly elicit counterarguments from them, change is unlikely.

> **The more patients verbalize their own desire and reasons for change, the more likely it is to happen.**

Mastering MI

MI is consistent with the idea of "patient activation"—getting people engaged in their own health care. It is also consistent with self-determination theory (Deci & Ryan, 2000). This involves tuning into them as people and calling forth what they see as important reasons to change, harnessing their own values, and showing faith in their ability to take even the smallest steps to better health. It also means offering advice and information that fits with what they think might be helpful.

It's like a dance, one where you move with people rather than against them, pointing them here and there in the interest of better health, while paying attention to how they respond to your efforts. In practice, as the many examples in this book will illustrate, MI involves a normal-sounding conversation, often simply allowing the patient to say why and how they might change.

The Six C's

We have found it helpful in training to offer learners a simple idea, the Six C's, to remind themselves about the ideal state of mind to be in when practicing MI:

> LET GO OF: Cleverness, Clutter, and Complexity
>
> HOLD ON TO: Compassion, Calm, and Curiosity
>
> AND: Point the conversation in the direction of change and show patients you believe the best answers are inside them.

Conclusion

MI is as much about what you don't do as what you do: When you ask a patient why they might change, you hold back from interrupting or stepping in with your views, and you call forth the language of change in a way that gives them, often for the first time, a chance to share with someone their heartfelt ideas for a healthier life. The skills involved are what we turn to in the next part of the book.

PART II

SKILLS

Speaking with dance teachers about learning to dance brings up some interesting parallels with improving clinical communication skills. They say that when learning the technical steps, tripping over your feet is part of the journey. You have to stumble a bit as you search for those fluid moments where everything seems to click into place. Both the steps and the overall feel of the dance must be kept in mind. If you have a partner, as in a tango, you also need to synchronize your movement with theirs. When you're leading, you learn how to gently follow and pay attention to how your partner responds. That's quite a lot to attend to.

Consultations are like dances: fluid, rich in potential, and with uncertain trajectories and outcomes. Working on core communication skills, which are the drivers of good practice, leads to those moments when what was once complex and a bit clumsy becomes much simpler and easier. We identify four specific skills that, once you acquire and refine them, make your consultations richer, more precise, and easier. You sit with a patient, ask a question (Chapter 3)—and because you know why you have asked it, your mind is free of distraction, and you are focused on the way they might respond, ready to listen, engage, and empower them. Then other skills besides questioning come into play (Chapters 4–6).

The four chapters that follow explore in depth each of these four core skills: open questions, listening statements, affirmations, and summaries. And, they include examples that illustrate how they are used in synchrony with one another. You are probably using versions of these skills in everyday practice already, and MI is about refining your use of these skills, a process that can continue throughout your career. In each chapter, we not only explore the basics, but we also clarify and illustrate how they are used in MI.

When practicing MI, the skills are used in a purposeful way, harnessed in the service of talking about the future, about change. For example, an open question about past failure is less likely to be helpful than one about future success. Not only are the skills focused on change, but their use also tends to form a pattern worth highlighting here before we dive into the detail: Thoughtfully selected open questions are used to encourage discussion about change, a bit like knocking on the door of someone's house. "What have you been doing or thinking about doing to stay healthy?" is a good example. If the patient responds and, in effect, opens the door, don't restrict yourself to a series of questions one after the other, but listen instead for a while before asking another question. Here, you will be best served by using listening statements and affirmations more than questions, while a summary is usually used toward the end of a sequence, to pull together the positive things you have heard.

The look and feel of an MI-inspired conversation are different from those of one governed by confrontation and disagreement. There will be fewer closed questions, many more curious open ones, and a good deal of listening, too. An MI trainer colleague, Kamilla Venner, put it this way: Practicing MI is like going into someone else's house. As she sees it, "[Their] world should be entered with respect, kindness, interest, and affirmation of what is good while refraining from offering advice about how to arrange the furniture" (Venner et al., 2007, p. 24). You are visiting patients' home territory, getting to see what they do and how they live their lives. It's both a privilege and a responsibility.

Will the use of these skills involve a degree of unlearning? If you have been schooled to ask short-answer questions as an expert problem-solver, then this part of the book will highlight the need to put some old questioning habits to one side and to be much more restrained with what you say to patients. The benefits are there for the taking.

CHAPTER 3

Asking

In the beginner's mind there are many possibilities,
but in the expert's there are few.
                                    —SHUNRYU SUZUKI

Your training will most likely have involved learning to ask a series of short-answer questions to patients, many of whom will expect this, especially if there is an acute problem that requires you to go down a decision tree to establish a provisional diagnosis.

This communication pattern has its limitations, the most obvious of which is the absence of human connection. Indeed, we have noticed that toward the end of their careers senior clinicians are using more open-ended questions that both engage the patient *and* provide rich detail for establishing a diagnosis. A second limitation is that, quite simply, many presenting problems, like back pain or tension headaches, do not have a single specific diagnosis. While you might want to rule out a less common diagnosis, you will soon gain tremendous value in a more open-ended approach to your assessment.

Much of health care these days deals with long-term conditions that are intertwined with patient behavior and lifestyle. The course and outcome of a chronic disease like diabetes are substantially determined by people's behavioral choices regarding such things as diet, physical activity, medication adherence, smoking, alcohol use, and health care visits (Steinberg & Miller, 2015). Providing health care under these circumstances is not as simple as asking questions and prescribing a remedy. What is really helpful is to pose questions to a *person* not just to a patient with a list of symptoms, to someone who needs to be involved in looking after their own health. What questions you ask and how you ask them can make all the difference to the progress of the consultation and its outcome.

Why Asking Matters

If your focus is on change in a patient's behavior and lifestyle, you have the advantage of another expert in the room. No one knows more about your patients than they do themselves, so to come up with the best plan, you tap their knowledge and expertise. How could a change in diet or exercise best fit into your patient's life? What would this person be ready, willing, and able to do?

By virtue of your training, you are probably well prepared to provide answers for patients, but health behavior change is a process of negotiation. Some patients want you to tell them what to do, and some will actually do what you suggest based on your advice alone. Physician advice to stop smoking, for example, can prompt 2–5% of smokers to quit, and more when it is accompanied by an offer to assist (Aveyard, Begh, Parsons, & West, 2012). The most common outcome of just telling people what to do, however, is that they will not do it, or may even do the opposite (de Almeida Neto, 2017; Dillard & Shen, 2005; Rains, 2013). It's a common frustration in health care and in parenting: "I tell them, and I tell them, and I tell them, and still they don't change." Sometimes the problem is the telling.

We suggest taking a little more time to *ask* rather than tell, to have a curious "beginner's mind" about how this patient might go about making health changes. After all, when talking about someone's life, it is more respectful to ask than to tell. By asking you can draw on patients' own wisdom and experience about themselves, and you don't have to come up with all of the answers yourself.

The Basics of Asking

The act of asking a question, particularly what we will describe as an open question, places a little responsibility on the person asked to answer. Allow enough time for that answer to come; don't feel obliged to speak if there have been a few seconds of silence.

Ask with genuine *curiosity*, with the humility that you don't already know the answer and the mindset that there are many possibilities. Inquiring about a patient's life, or their perspective on their presenting problems, is not at all like a cross-examining attorney who wants to elicit a predetermined answer. When you ask with genuine curiosity, *you don't know* how this patient might respond, let alone address changes in their health habits. The patient may not yet know, either. Be curious together.

Open Questions

Most health care providers are accustomed to asking closed questions, to which there is a short answer: "yes" or "no," where it hurts, when it started, or how much pain on a 10-point scale. Open questions give the patient a much wider field of possible answers. It's not binary or multiple choice. Most likely you already do ask some open questions:

- "How have you been feeling lately?"
- "What has changed since the last time I saw you?"
- "How has your family responded to this?"
- "Tell me about the physical activity or exercise you are doing."

The last of these is phrased as an imperative statement, but it is still essentially a question, an open invitation to tell you more.

If, like many providers, you work on a tight schedule, you may feel hesitant to ask open questions, and indeed it's up to you to decide how best to spend your time. Keep in mind that the disadvantage of just going down a list of closed questions is what you *don't* learn. Sometimes just a couple of open questions elicit the answers the closed questions you might have used would have, *and* will also reveal important information that you might otherwise have missed. Patients additionally appreciate the opportunity to tell you a bit more. When you use open questions, patients can even feel as though you have spent more time with them than you actually have because of the quality of your listening to their responses.

> **When you use open questions, patients can feel you spent more time with them than you actually did.**

CONSIDER: A Stone Wall

Change is hard, for us and for our patients. Often we know what we need to do, but the aggregate of all of it can look insurmountable. Patients' resistance often seems like a dam, a huge stone wall, too large for me to take down. But then it occurred to me that maybe I didn't have to take down the whole wall; maybe all I needed to do was take down one or two stones from the top and let the water do the rest.

Motivational interviewing is about finding that one stone which, when moved, breaches the resistance, releasing change, a little at first, but growing with time. How often have I asked about that colonoscopy? Perhaps if I asked a little differently, spending just a little more time now, it would get done. And I wouldn't have to ask again for 10 years. And I might save a life. How powerful is that?

—Cleve Sharp, MD

Asking and MI

Asking in MI is guided by which of the four processes you feel are most relevant at the time. As you will see in the examples below, they are all focused on change.

Engaging

Open questions in the midst of the engagement process are used to establish or reestablish *connection*. They are not necessarily directly about change but simply help you and the patient share an understanding of how they are feeling.

In MI most questions are focused on change.

- "How are you feeling today?"
- "What matters the most for you right now?"
- "How can I help?"

Focusing

These open questions are used to *establish direction*, to clarify a topic or goal you will be talking about.

- "What change in lifestyle might we most usefully focus on?"
- "How do you feel about us talking about getting a vaccination?"
- "I wonder about your use of alcohol, but how do you feel about talking about this?"

Evoking

In the evoking process, open questions are used to *invite change talk* and give the patient opportunity to wonder aloud in your presence why and how change might come about. You ask *particular* questions (which are still open questions) that invite your patient to voice the arguments for change, rather than you doing so. You will notice there is a rich diversity here, and the questions often have a hypothetical quality; in other words, they simply encourage the patient to imagine, without any pressure to make a decision of some kind. Some questions focus on the *why* of change, someone's *desire*, their *reasons* to change or the *need* to do something different. Others might focus on the *how*, their confidence in their *ability* to change.

> **Ask questions that invite your patient to voice the arguments for change.**

- "How might your life be different if you made this change?" (Desire)
- "What good might come from decreasing your alcohol use?" (Reasons)
- "What concerns you the most about your weight at the moment?" (Need)
- "If you did decide to decrease your drinking, how might you go about it?" (Ability)

Planning

These open question are used to evoke ideas from the patient about what a plan might look like, to help them *narrow down* the possibilities. They are best used when the patient is ready to make a change.

- "So what do you think you might do?"
- "What are some positive steps you would be willing to try?"
- "Of these different possible changes we've discussed, which one seems like a good place to start?"

Rather than trying to insert motivation or action in your patients, asking such open questions is a way to evoke their own willingness and ideas.

Asking in Everyday Practice

PRACTITIONER: So, just to sum up what I've said so far: Your lab test shows that you have an unusual amount of sugar circulating in your bloodstream. We could call it type 2 diabetes or predia-betes, but either way you can do some things to stay healthy and avoid long-term complications. What are you thinking you might do at this point?

PATIENT: Well, I certainly didn't expect to get bad news today. I've been feeling fine.

PRACTITIONER: In what ways do you think of this as bad news?

PATIENT: I guess I think you're telling me that I have to change the way I eat in order to stay healthy.

PRACTITIONER: What you decide to do about this is really up to you, but let me ask you this. What do you need your health for?

PATIENT: What?

PRACTITIONER: I'm asking why it's important for you to be healthy. What does your good health allow you to do?

PATIENT: I kind of take my health for granted. I mean, I've always been a healthy and energetic person. I wouldn't want to lose that. I want to stay healthy for my family, too.

In a conversation like this, you would normally be using more than one skill. Asking would be interwoven with listening, affirming, and summarizing skills that build on each other. In subsequent chapters we add these skills one by one and show how they can be combined. This dialogue is focused on asking. The interviewer asks several open questions, the answers to which are likely to be change talk:

- "What are you thinking you might do at this point?"
- "In what ways do you think of this as bad news?"
- "What do you need your health for? What does your good health allow you to do?"

Even if the only tool you had were asking open questions, this dialogue is already moving in the right direction.

TRY THIS

1. The next time you are sitting with a patient for whom health behavior change is important, try asking instead of telling. Why would the patient want to make a change? What ideas do they have for beginning steps? From your patient's perspective, what are the best reasons to make a change? How important is it to do so, and why?

2. How could you change these closed questions into open questions?

> Closed question: "Would you like to lose some weight?"
>
> Your open question: _____
>
> Another suggestion: "What would be the advantages of losing some weight?"
>
> Closed question: "How about trying an antidepressant medication?"
>
> Your open question: _____
>
> Another suggestion: "How do you feel about taking an antidepressant medication?"
>
> Closed question: "Can you get some exercise before I see you next time?"
>
> Your open question: _____
>
> Another suggestion: "What sort of exercise might you get before I see you next time?"

Asking is only one skill. What do you do after you ask a question? In the next chapter, we explain a second skill that blends well with asking—a particular kind of listening.

CHAPTER 4

Listening

Without listening, speaking no longer heals.
—HENRI NOUWEN

Listening is a big subject, deeply embedded in literature, psychology, and therapy, and one truth that emerges is that listening with empathy is a naturally healing process. The Chinese character for listening, for example, includes five elements: the ears (to hear), the eyes (to see), the mind (to think), undivided attention (to focus), and the heart (to feel).

Listening in MI involves particular attention to your use of the spoken word as a vehicle for transmitting empathy. It is certainly not a matter of sitting back and keeping quiet or letting the consultation run wild and free. The use of listening in MI comes from the world of counseling, where it is seen as both an attitude and a technique. In MI listening is used to engage and connect as well as to evoke a person's motivation to change.

You may think of good listening as just keeping quiet, and compared to doing all the talking yourself, there is definitely a role for some silence. The skill of listening on which we focus in this chapter, however, is quite active. It requires paying close attention, searching for meaning, and conveying your understanding back to the patient. There is strong research evidence for the value of this particular kind of listening in helping relationships, within and beyond health care (Elliot, Bohart, Watson, & Murphy, 2018; Gordon & Edwards, 1997; Rakel, 2018). In this book, we use the

Listening requires paying close attention and conveying your understanding back to the patient.

term "listening statement" when discussing this act of conveying your understanding back to the patient.

It does take time to listen, but the kind of listening we are talking about here can also save you time—and misunderstanding. A conversation often moves faster and farther when you listen skillfully. Similarly to asking open questions, listening also allows you to learn important things that you otherwise could have missed. Many people who go into helping professions do so, at least in part, because they enjoy meeting people. With time pressures being what they are in health care, the kind of listening we argue for makes it possible to have a more meaningful conversation that lets you establish a quicker and deeper connection with those you serve.

> A conversation moves faster and farther when you listen skillfully.

We describe the essence of skillful listening as "mirroring." Using a listening statement, you reflect back to patients how you understand their meaning, often going a bit beyond the words they have spoken to venture a guess about what they might mean. This technique has also been called active, or reflective, or empathic listening. It entails much more than simply repeating what you heard, and you can get better at it with practice.

Why Listening Matters

An obvious benefit of good listening is that you get a more accurate understanding of the patient and the circumstances surrounding their presenting problem. This understanding is important in collecting basic information about symptoms, but even more so in developing a trusting relationship with your patients. To listen well conveys respect: "What you say matters to me, and I want to be sure I understand." In the course of a typical week, how many minutes do you experience someone listening to you with no agenda other than to understand what you mean or feel? Giving someone an empathic listening ear, even for a short time, is a compassionate gift.

A skillful healer quickly establishes a working alliance with patients. The same treatment procedures can have very different outcomes depending on who provides them, and how. This has been known for a long time in psychotherapy, that the therapist's stance and manner often matter more than the specific treatment being used. There are particular skills that render healers more effective (Miller & Moyers, 2021). Of these skills, empathic listening has perhaps the strongest evidence base (Elliott et al., 2018; Miller, 2018; Rakel, 2018).

The Basics of Listening

Think about a single communication. Before the speaker says a word, there is a meaning to be conveyed. The speaker puts that meaning into words, which is the first place communication can go wrong because people don't necessarily say what they mean. Next, you have to hear the words correctly, and mishearing is a second potential pitfall. Having heard the words, you have to decode what they mean. Thus, even with a single communication, there are three places where misunderstanding can occur: sending, receiving, and decoding. Most of us assume the meaning we make of the words we think we hear is actually what the person meant. With so much potential for the intended meaning to be missed, we need to be more discerning about how we listen.

One good way to clarify communication is to compare your understanding with the speaker's meaning. A simple but awkward way to do this is to keep asking, "Is this what you mean?" But, there is a better way.

Listening Statements

A time-tested (and research-tested) alternative is to offer back to the person what we mentioned earlier, a short summary of what you understood, which we refer to as a "listening statement." You are in essence serving as a mirror to reflect meaning, and in the process, you and the patient can together develop a clearer understanding. But, you need to be skillful in doing this. A simple reflection, just repeating what the person said with minimal change, is easy but limiting, and can leave you getting nowhere or going around in circles.

PATIENT: I don't feel well.

PRACTITIONER: You're not feeling well.

PATIENT: No, I don't feel good.

PRACTITIONER: Not so good today.

PATIENT: No.

A better form of reflecting what a patient says makes use of a listening statement, wherein you venture a *guess* about what the person *means*. You play back what the patient said, but in a somewhat different way to see whether your understanding is accurate.

PATIENT: I don't feel well.

PRACTITIONER: You're in pain. [*A reasonable guess from the patient's appearance*]

PATIENT: Yes, my stomach hurts, and I also feel sick.

PRACTITIONER: Sick to your stomach, nauseous. [*Another guess*]

PATIENT: Yes exactly, and I don't know why.

It actually doesn't matter if you guess wrong in the beginning. Either way people will tell you more about what they *do* mean.

In this simple illustration, you could do as well just by asking, "Tell me what you're feeling." It's when the conversation gets into more sensitive territory, and particularly when you are talking about health behavior change, that mirroring is better than asking. Why is that?

Suppose a patient has alluded to some marital difficulties. Look at two possible responses, which are different only in what you do with your voice. In the first, your voice rises at the end to make it a question. In the second, your voice tone drops at the end, making it a statement. Try saying them aloud:

"You and your husband aren't getting along?"

"You and your husband aren't getting along."

Can you feel the difference? It's subtle, but making your response a question can put a person on the defensive. As we said in Chapter 3, asking a question places pressure on the person to answer. By contrast, the same words expressed as a statement flow like a conversation. It may feel odd to you at first because you're aware that you are making a guess, but try it. Our experience is that mirroring statements are received more comfortably and help the patient talk to you more honestly than responses phrased as questions.

Listening and MI

In MI, this foundational skill of listening statements is taken a step further, to using them in a purposeful manner to focus on change and help patients to break free of ambivalence. To begin with, in the start-up processes of engaging and focusing, asking and empathic listening may be all you need to do. Then when it comes to evoking and planning, you can use listening statements strategically.

Listening is used to help patients break through ambivalence.

As discussed in Chapter 3, one strategy is to ask open questions, the answer to which is likely to be change talk: desire, ability, reasons, and need for change. When you hear change talk, offer a listening statement.

Thus, patients hear themselves voicing change talk when you have asked for it, then they hear it again as you mirror it. That's what we mean by using listening in a strategic manner, and you will see this illustrated shortly. This way of carrying on the conversation not only strengthens the change talk, but also is likely to evoke still more of it (Apodaca et al., 2016; Villarosa-Hurlocker, O'Sickey, Houck, & Moyers, 2019).

Another common use of listening statements in MI is in response to patient sustain talk or discord. This may seem counterintuitive, but mirroring a "resistive" statement lets the patient know that you have heard and understand them—as you will see in the example below. The temptation is to disagree and persuade with such statements, but doing that tends only to entrench a patient's reluctance to change. Resist the common urge ("righting reflex") to push back against and try to correct sustain talk. It's a struggle you are unlikely to win.

Mirroring sustain talk lets the patient know you have heard and understand them.

CONSIDER: From the Frontline

By engaging a patient through listening, the possibility of frustration between patients and providers disappears. Instead, both parties are working in sync to achieve shared goals, resulting in a positive and rewarding outcome for both patients and providers. Learning motivational interviewing allowed me to reconnect with the reason I chose a career in medicine. Through utilizing this method, I witnessed firsthand immense progress with patients that traditionally would have been considered "difficult." After experiencing the power of this approach, I couldn't fathom returning to the traditional, paternalistic approach to patient care.

—MARA RICE-STUBBS, MD

Listening in Everyday Practice

This dialogue with a patient newly diagnosed with prediabetic metabolic syndrome picks up from where it left off in Chapter 3, having begun with a few open questions.

PRACTITIONER: I'm asking why it's important for you to be healthy. What does your good health allow you to do?

PATIENT: I kind of take my health for granted. I mean, I've always been a healthy and energetic person. I wouldn't want to lose that. I want to stay healthy for my family, too.

PRACTITIONER: You're accustomed to being healthy, and that's important for you and your family.

PATIENT: Yes! As you know, we have two young daughters. I enjoy playing soccer with them, and I want to be there for them as they become adults.

PRACTITIONER: It feels good to you to be able to keep up with them.

PATIENT: When I can. I know I could stand to lose some weight.

PRACTITIONER: That might help you on the soccer field, and it's also a good idea in managing your blood sugar. Why else is your health important to you?

PATIENT: I dream about grandchildren—not too soon, mind you!

PRACTITIONER: You can imagine it, the fun of grandchildren.

PATIENT: I do think about it once the girls are grown. I like having kids around. Of course, it's up to them.

PRACTITIONER: I wonder what you know or what you've heard about what people with this metabolic syndrome can do to stay healthy.

PATIENT: Like I said, lose some weight. I eat fairly healthy already, but I suppose I could make some changes there.

PRACTITIONER: You can see some things you could change there.

PATIENT: I do have a sweet tooth. But you know, I've been feeling fine, and this was just one lab test, right?

PRACTITIONER: It puzzles you how this could be happening while you still feel fine.

PATIENT: I mean, I guess it's good to catch things like this early. I just don't know how seriously to take it.

PRACTITIONER: You wonder if it's worth making changes at this point because you're not experiencing any real health problems so far.

PATIENT: I don't want to have health problems. My health is important to me.

Look back through the practitioner's responses. Beyond a few open questions, every response is a listening statement (or "reflection"), offering a short summary of what the patient was saying. The first reflection did more than repeat, by including something that had not quite been said: "You're accustomed to being healthy, *and that's important for you and your family.*" It wasn't a big jump from the patient's own words, but it did what we call "lending" change talk. It offered a possible change talk statement about importance, which the patient accepted.

Part way through, a listening statement is followed by an open question: "Why else is your health important to you?" The interviewer is evoking a list of the patient's own motivations for change, and more change talk follows: grandchildren. Then another open question: "I wonder what you know or what you've heard about what people with this metabolic syndrome can do to stay healthy." It invites the patient to a planning process—what changes might help to control blood sugar.

Finally, some doubt emerges: How serious is this, really? The interviewer responds to two instances of sustain talk with listening statements: "It puzzles you . . ." and "You wonder if. . . ." Had the interviewer argued that the problem is serious, the likely result would be more sustain talk. Instead, the reflections are followed by more change talk.

Every time you make one listening statement you get immediate feedback from your patient about its accuracy. Each time you also learn a bit more, which means that you have more to reflect. Once mirroring becomes easier, you can try using it strategically. It *matters* what you reflect. Listen in particular for any change talk, and mirror it back. Pay attention to what your patient says *next* when you reflect change talk. Most often it is more change talk, and that matters. When MI is going well, you are helping patients to talk themselves into making healthy behavior changes. Part of them already wants to do so. It's like there is a committee inside them, deciding whether to invest in change. Some members see reasons for change and think it may be time to do so. You are helping those members of the committee to speak up.

Particularly when you feel the righting reflex—the urge to disagree, correct, fix, and give advice—consider mirroring instead. (We come back to advice giving in Chapter 11.) Mirroring doesn't always work, but it's surprising how often you free up your patients' "better angels" to fly.

TRY THIS

1. Write down three to four things you often hear from patients that frustrate or discourage you. Then for each one, come up with a listening statement you could offer instead of what you might ordinarily say. How do you think a patient might respond?

PATIENT: _____

Listening statement: _____

PATIENT: _____

Listening statement: _____

PATIENT: _____

Listening statement: _____

2. Here are some patient statements that contain both change talk and sustain talk. Try to come up with a listening statement (not a question) for each one that focuses on the change talk, rather than the sustain talk.

PATIENT: I know I ought to stop smoking, but it's the only way I have to relax.

Listening statement: _____

PATIENT: I would like to take off some weight, but I've tried several diets and I can't keep it off.

Listening statement: _____

PATIENT: I've heard that these vaccines can make you sick later on. I want to stay healthy, but I don't like taking something I don't really need.

Listening statement: _____

CHAPTER 5

Affirming

When you're that young, it doesn't take a lot to be encouraged,
or discouraged. . . . They raised my game . . . they saw something
in me I didn't see in myself.

—Sir Ken Robinson

The skill of affirming is perhaps the least appreciated in health care. It is a form of encouragement that allows you to tap a person's reserves of well-being and hope for the future, whatever challenges they are facing. The technique involves highlighting what you notice about their strengths and efforts, and pointing this out to them. It is a statement that you make to the patient, and it can even be used in the face of apparent failure. It offers hope to patients and improves trust in you like few other techniques.

Why Affirming Matters

When a person feels affirmed, it helps them to recognize their existing strengths and positive qualities in consultations that are all too often focused only on this or that problem. They might have come for help with a complaint of some kind, and here is a practitioner who sees more than just a diagnosis or list of symptoms. Affirming helps patients to rise up to the challenges they are facing. Indeed, there's a body of research on what happens when people affirm themselves; it appears to make them feel less defensive and more accepting of information that is potentially threatening (Sherman & Cohen, 2006). Self-affirmation can apparently also impact weight loss (Logel & Cohen, 2012) and adherence to medication (Wileman et al., 2014). Offering an affirmation to a patient is likely to have a similar uplifting effect, and if you are focusing on behavior change, patients are likely to start talking about this with increasing motivation and commitment. It takes very little time and can changes lives, which is what Sir Ken Robinson was pointing out in the opening quote for this chapter.

Is affirming different from praise? Here, it can be helpful to imagine a continuum: At the one end is praise, a positive comment or judgment you make about a person's efforts ("Great, you did it"). Around the middle are compliments like "I appreciate how well you have managed your blood pressure." At the top end are affirmations, deeper comments on a person's strengths and enduring qualities. Patients often respond differently to each of these forms of encouragement. They may dismiss superficial praise as disingenuous, or feel judged by you. Deeper affirming tends to encourage patients to say more about their own positive qualities and efforts, even when struggling to cope (Miller & Moyers, 2021). Noticing how patients react is important when offering any of these forms of encouragement.

The Basics of Affirming

Affirming is not a complex technique requiring time-consuming effort or specialist training. It often just involves noticing what's right there in front of you. Here's quite a striking example.

CONSIDER: The Power of Affirmation

As he left I remember shaking his hand and spontaneously pointing out to him that he was a dignified person in the face of all these troubles. He was living in poverty, he had Type I diabetes, and he was about to undergo assessment for the amputation of one of his legs. He was dependent on multiple substances, and beer was his favorite. I noticed the dignity in the immaculate suit he was wearing, and I commented on it. Even his walking stick had a gold handle.

When he returned a week later he announced, "I stopped smoking, thank you. It was something you said last time. . . . You told me I was a dignified guy, so I walked out and thought, 'That's right, no one can take this away from me, and I'm going to use my dignity to show those doctors a thing or two,' so I stopped smoking there and then."

—Stephen Rollnick

The affirmation ("You are a dignified person") seemed to shine a light on something about him that in his own words, "no one can take away from me"—that is, a personal strength. Affirming was the act of pointing out that strength to him, like holding up a mirror for him to look into. Then he encouraged himself to quit smoking. The word "encourage" connotes how affirmation might work: You help patients face their situation with the courage they already have inside them.

Affirming involves noticing what's in front of you.

Affirming highlights a patient's strengths, values, achievements, or efforts. Notice how the word "I" is usually absent from an affirmation. It is not a judgment you are handing down to the patient, like "I'm proud of you," but simply a statement of fact about something you observe in them. For example:

> "Despite all these setbacks, you decided to get here to this appointment."
>
> "You are determined to get on top of this condition."
>
> "Being a good mom to your kids is important to you."

As troubled as patients may seem, their strengths often lie just beneath the surface of their talk about problems. They bring a range of qualities to the table: flexibility, focus, perseverance, organization, motivation, generosity, bravery, selflessness, resilience, positivity, calm, and caring—the list can be doubled quite easily. With an affirmation, you tell patients about such a quality that you notice in them.

Affirming highlights a patient's strengths, values, or efforts.

Forming an Affirmation

To offer an affirmation, try out three practices:

1. *Put the strengths lenses on.* We use the idea of lenses here to suggest that while you can and must notice problems (deficit lenses), it can transform your practice to flick a second lens over the first one, filtered for seeing positive strengths and achievements. You get used to noticing positive qualities and behavior, and affirmations are really just the verbal expression and natural consequence of looking for strengths.

2. *Make a statement that highlights enduring positive qualities.* Offer a statement about the strengths you recognize, as succinctly as you

can, and then allow the patient to take the conversation forward. This is the moment when you may notice uplift in their pride, morale, and motivation.

3. *Ask a curious question about their strengths or effort, then highlight the reply with an affirmation.* You can ask an interested question that invites them to talk about their strengths, making it easy for you to offer an affirmation by way of listening statements. For example, to a young person with diabetes, the question "How did you manage to do that?" might elicit a reply like, "I took a deep breath and said, 'No thanks, I'll keep off the sweets tonight.'" Then it is a straight-forward matter to offer an affirmation like "Your determination came to the fore." The conversation will unfold, often with further uplifting talk from the patient, like "I get like that, I see things really clearly and it feels good." Affirmation is simple to deliver, with rich rewards if used with care, compassion, and skill.

> **Affirmations are the natural consequence of looking for strengths.**

Modest Use, Better Progress

Both patients and the cultures they live in vary in the use of and responses to encouragement. Affirmations are more widely used in North America, for example, much less so in the United Kingdom and Scandinavian countries. Patients will also vary over time in their response to affirmation. For example, an affirmation might be hard for someone to accept when they are feeling low, and could come across as inauthentic and even unhelpful. The value of using MI and skills like affirming lies in your ability to sense how patients are reacting.

> **Affirmation is simple to deliver, with rich rewards.**

Affirming and MI

When you are talking about change, the use of affirming highlights the values, strengths, and behavior that might bring this about. Affirming examples include: "Despite everything, you made this appointment wanting to get this sorted out." "You seem to know what's best for you." "When you make up your mind, you usually mean it." Or, "Being a good dad is important to you." The patient is likely to elaborate on your observation, often in the form of change talk. Consider this brief example:

PRACTITIONER: What ideas do you have about how you might lose weight?

PATIENT: Not many. I'm so busy and I can't see a way through, but I have been thinking about it. [*Change talk*]

PRACTITIONER: Even though life is really busy, you are still finding the time to give it some thought. [*Affirming*]

PATIENT: Yes, it's frustrating because I know, just like I did with stopping smoking, that there's got to be a way of losing weight. [*Change talk*]

PRACTITIONER: There's your determination again. [*Affirming*] You are searching for a way to do it.

PATIENT: Exactly, I must find a way. [*Change talk*]

Searching for strengths pulls you into seeing the patient as a unique individual with their own special brand of courage and other qualities that can make a difference in achieving better health. It's often more enjoyable to view patients this way because instead of feeling the need to solve problems for them, you work on bringing out the best in them. Some research teams have studied this in depth, by counting the use of skills like listening statements and affirmation, and whether they are followed by the kind of change talk likely to predict actual behavior change. One recent study concluded, "Affirm[ing] was the only . . . [practitioner] behavior that both increased change talk and also reduced sustain talk" (Apodaca et al., 2016).

Affirming in Everyday Practice

Imagine that common scenario in which talk about problems comes tumbling out of the patient. What you want is to turn the conversation around and look positively to the future. Affirming is sometimes just the tool for lifting someone out of problem talk.

PRACTITIONER: How might you find a way through all these pressures and take even just the first one or two steps to feeling healthier? [*An open guiding question about change*]

PATIENT: Hah. (*Laughs in resignation.*) Now you are asking. I get this disease, then I lose my job, just like that, out of the blue, we have no damn money and then they say I must lose weight and get more exercise. Any more pressures, hey? (*Laughs again.*)

PRACTITIONER: Your sense of humor certainly helps. [*Affirmation*]

PATIENT: Otherwise, I'd fall apart to be honest, I got to stay positive but really, how can I now start losing weight? Give me a break, won't you. [*Sustain talk*]

PRACTITIONER: Laughter only gets you so far, and it's your courage that's needed somehow. [*Affirmation*]

PATIENT: Seriously now, you are right. Some courage I'm going to need. [*Change talk*]

TRY THIS

1. Transform simple praise into affirmation: This exercise challenges you to hold back for a moment when you want to superficially praise a patient and instead transform your good intention into a deeper affirmation. We make the transformation in the first example, then provide you with two to practice for yourself:

   Praise: "Oh, that's excellent, well done for taking that first step."

   Deeper affirmation: "You made a decision, and your determination got you there."

   Praise: "You want to try to take the tablets more regularly. That's really good."

   Deeper affirmation: _____

   Another possible affirmation: "You have given this some serious thought before coming down here today."

   Praise: "That's such good progress to lose a few pounds like that."

   Deeper affirmation: _____

   Another possible affirmation: "Once you made that decision, you stuck to it."

2. Affirm even in the face of failure: Here are three examples of producing an affirmation when a patient is talking about their difficulties. We then provide you with two examples for you to try out yourself. Remember that affirming is not some kind of verbal trick, but a genuine expression of your interest in the patient's

qualities and efforts. They get to see their struggles and apparent failures as opportunities to do better next time. You'll notice this in the change talk that follows the affirmations you provide.

PATIENT: I don't know. . . . I just never seem to succeed, no matter how hard I try.

PRACTITIONER: You're not someone who wants to give up on this. [*Affirming*]

PATIENT: No, I only wish I could find a way. [*Change talk*]

PATIENT: I went home and kept off the sweets all day, for two days, and then I got stressed and BANG . . . it all went downhill because I gave in and went for the chocolates again, and I felt so bad.

PRACTITIONER: It's been up and down, and you've come here today determined to find a way through. [*Affirming*]

PATIENT: Thanks, and I still want to make progress. I must. [*Change talk*]

PATIENT: She goes off to work and leaves me with the kids, and it's not that easy.

PRACTITIONER: You strive to be a good dad whatever the struggles you face. [*Affirming*]

PATIENT: Yes, I work hard on being there for the kids.

PRACTITIONER: You have come down to this clinic many times over the years, and you have been looking for a solution to this problem.

PATIENT: I only wish I could get rid of this pain, but I can't.

Your affirmation: _____

Another possible affirmation: "Leading a normal and active life is really important to you."

PRACTITIONER: This has been a big upset for you at the school because you feel they are treating your child unfairly.

PATIENT: I went down there and told them they can't treat my kid like that at school.

Your affirmation: _____

Another possible affirmation: "You stuck to your principles and decided to sort this out."

Once you get the hang of the basics of affirming, you can polish your skills in everyday conversations. Children, for example, lap up affirmation, as do adults in practically any walk of life. We view it not just as an attitude toward people, but also a skill that you can get better at.

CHAPTER 6

Summarizing

Life is the first gift, love is the second,
and understanding the third.
—MARGE PIERCY

If you take your understanding of what the patient has said and share this with them, it can be powerful and helpful, whether you get this information exactly right or not. Your genuine desire to capture their experience is what really matters. You create a shared understanding.

As described in Chapter 4, a listening statement is a short summary of what you think your patient means. It's usually more than repetition, and includes a guess about what the person *might* mean. When you practice making listening statements, over time you receive immediate feedback from patients about whether your guess was correct, and so you gradually get better at guessing people's hidden meaning from their words, posture, and facial cues.

In this chapter, we describe a fourth basic skill beyond asking, listening, and affirming. It is summarizing what you've heard over a span of time, like a collection of listening statements strung together, and it matters *what* you put into such a summary. After even 5 minutes of talking with a patient, you may have heard quite a bit if you're listening well, so what should you include in a summary, and why?

Why Summarizing Matters

What patients say does matter, and you significantly influence what they say. First they hear what they themselves say. Then they hear it again as you offer a listening statement. Now with a summary, they may hear it for yet a third time.

When you offer a summary, you are shining a light on certain aspects of what was said, presumably those details you regard as most important. In essence, you are encouraging the patient to listen again to what they said. Notice that in MI, it is not a summary of what *you* have said. It is what patients themselves say that is most likely to have an impact on their motivation to change.

Summarizing also conveys respect. It communicates, "What you tell me is so important that I remember it." By the way, when you listen well to patients, they are also more likely to listen to you.

Summaries also *pull together* important content. For example, you may hear various kinds of change talk scattered through what a patient says and interspersed with its opposite, sustain talk. That's normal when people are ambivalent. It can have more impact for patients to hear all of their own change talk collected together in a summary. There's just something about hearing a *re-collection* of your own words.

Finally, making a summary allows you to change the subject with a patient on board. Indeed, we know one practitioner who described her learning about the summary as a revelation of sorts: "Until I learned to summarise, I could never really find a way to politely call a halt to a patient speaking. Now, I ask permission to summarise, and when the patient hears in the summary that I have been listening he or she is more than happy for me to talk about something else."

When you listen well, patients are more likely to listen to you.

The Basics of Summarizing

No doubt, you already use summaries in your regular practice. When you're finishing a visit with a patient, it's common to pull together the key pieces of what you have said. "So, it looks like what you have is a virus, not a bacterial infection, and so an antibiotic won't help here unfortunately. I have suggested you take lots of liquids and use aspirin to keep your temperature down. If this doesn't clear up fairly soon, or gets worse, please get back in touch with us. Do you have any questions?"

The kind of summarizing used in MI is a bit different; it pulls together things that the *patient* has said. Probably you already do some of this as well, for example, when you first ask patients about their symptoms. "You're having some trouble sleeping; you usually get to sleep okay, but then you wake up in the wee hours and don't fall back asleep.

You said you feel tired most of the time and don't enjoy doing things that you used to like. You've also lost some weight. What else do you notice?"

The basics of this kind of summarizing are fairly simple. You remember things your patient has told you, and you gather them together like flowers in a bouquet. Notice that the summaries often end with an open or closed question like "What else?" or "Did I get that right?" Pull together things you have heard while listening, and ask a question.

> Gather together things your patient has told you, like flowers in a bouquet.

Summarizing and MI

But, *what* things? Of all that a patient has told you, what should you put in your summary? It depends whether you're engaging, focusing, evoking, or planning. During the engaging process, you may be listening to what your patient is experiencing, pulling it together in a clinical picture. In focusing, you may be assembling a list of concerns and clarifying which need to be addressed the most. When evoking, you listen for and collect patients' change talk. Finally, when planning, you might collect the various possible courses of action and what the patient has told you about each of them.

Summaries may mark the end of one task as a transition to the next. "So if I understand you right, what is most important to you is to regain your mobility, to get back on your feet, and be able to take walks again like you enjoy. The pain in your hip and back has been the biggest obstacle lately, and you're hoping for relief from that pain. You mentioned, too, that you would prefer not to have to use a cane. So, shall we talk about how best to get you back to walking again?" This is an example of a transition into planning. Mini-summaries can also be used along the way as you are collecting content. "So far you have told me about your fatigue and about the stress at work. What else?"

Summarizing in Everyday Practice

Here is an example of how MI can be used when you are evoking a patient's own motivation for change. This is one of the most common uses of MI, and can support patient activation for involvement in their own health promotion (Hibbard, Mahoney, Stock, & Tusler, 2007; Moore, Wolever, Hibbard, & Lawson, 2012). Here, you are asking open questions to evoke change talk, then reflecting, affirming, and summarizing what you hear.

PRACTITIONER: Could I ask what you are thinking about smoking at this point? [*Open question, asking permission*]

PATIENT: Yeah, I'm still smoking cigarettes. I don't need you to tell me it's not good for me.

PRACTITIONER: You already know. [*Listening statement*]

PATIENT: Who doesn't know these days? My kids are always bugging me to stop.

PRACTITIONER: I know they're important to you. What worries them? [*Affirmation, listening statement*]

PATIENT: They say, "I don't want you to die, Daddy."

PRACTITIONER: Ouch! They're really worried. What do you yourself think? [*Listening statement, open question*]

PATIENT: I don't want to get lung cancer like my mother did.

PRACTITIONER: So, you've seen that firsthand. What else do you know about smoking and health? [*Listening statement, open question to evoke change talk*]

PATIENT: Bad for your heart?

PRACTITIONER: Sure is. It's the biggest cause of preventable death. [*Providing information*]

PATIENT: Really.

PRACTITIONER: And, how has smoking been a hassle for you? What have you noticed? [*Open question to evoke change talk*]

PATIENT: It gets more expensive all the time.

PRACTITIONER: Uh-huh. You're spending more. What else? [*Listening statement, open question*]

PATIENT: I don't know. People look at you when you smoke and cough sometimes, with like disapproval or disgust.

PRACTITIONER: You imagine what they're thinking. [*Listening statement*]

PATIENT: It's pretty clear sometimes on their face, or they say things.

PRACTITIONER: So, the cost and disapproval. What else have you noticed? [*Mini-summary, open question*]

PATIENT: Well, I've told you that I can get out of breath climbing stairs.

PRACTITIONER: You've been thinking about this a lot. It costs more to keep smoking, and you feel social disapproval. Your children are worrying about losing you, and you know about cancer and heart disease risks. In fact, you had firsthand experience of that in your family. You've noticed that you get out of breath easily, and you mentioned coughing. When you look at all that, what are you thinking at this point? [*Summary statement transitioning into planning*]

In this 2-minute conversation, the clinician has heard several change talk themes, and pulls them together in a summary and then asks an open question that might open the door for planning. It's not often that smokers keep talking about reasons for change with a good listener, then hear their own change talk pulled together in a bouquet. It's an unusual and potentially persuasive experience. It's not that you are persuading them; they are actually persuading themselves, by virtue of how you arrange the conversation.

Where might this conversation go from here? The clinician could decide that what has been discussed is enough for now and let it percolate within the patient. The conversation so far was mostly about reasons, and the dialogue could continue with open questions about ability, importance, or desire for change. Depending on how the patient responds, they might discuss when and how to quit, still honoring the patient's autonomy of choice. There is a lot of flexibility with this set of clinical skills, and the discussion doesn't have to take very long.

Summaries help in evoking a patient's own motivation for change.

TRY THIS

1. **Private rehearsal.** Imagine you're consulting with a patient, and what is needed is a change in the person's behavior or lifestyle. Pick a health behavior issue that is common in your practice. If you asked open questions about desire, ability, reasons, and need for change, what might a patient tell you? List them in your mind or on paper and then pull them together in a summary of the patient's own motivations for change.

2. **Recall key words.** When you are asking a patient open questions that evoke change talk, try to remember what they are telling you, then pull it together in a summary. A colleague once put it this way: "As I listen to the patient, I hang up the key words or phrases they use on pegs in my mind. Then when it is time to summarize, I pull these down off the pegs."

3. **Leave off the extra words.** When you summarize, make it as lean as possible. Try to avoid a lengthy introduction like "One thing I would like to do now is summarize what you have said and point out what I have noticed because these things are important and if you think about it. . . ." There's no need for most of these words, especially the word "I."

PART III

MOTIVATIONAL INTERVIEWING IN PRACTICE

Imagine there is a friendly coach who sits on your shoulder in consultations, acting as your wise guide, and they quietly ask you to stop, and whisper in your ear, "Tell me, *why* are you doing what you are doing?"

The aim of this part of the book is to help you answer that question, aware that conversations don't go in straight lines, and that all sorts of currents can swing them this way and that. The four-processes model of MI practice (see Miller & Rollnick, 2013), which provides the structure for the next four chapters, is designed to help you answer the coach's question.

- "I'm trying to establish a good relationship," or "I noticed the patient resisting so I am backing off and reestablishing connection"—these answers tell you that you are working on the *engaging* process (Chapter 7).

- "I'm checking to see whether the patient is happy to talk about quitting smoking rather than getting more exercise," or "I'm not sure exactly what change we might be talking about, so I thought I would check this with the patient first." These answers mean you are working on the *focusing* process (Chapter 8).

- "I'm wanting to let the patient tell me why losing weight is a good idea," or "I'm handing it over to him to talk about the benefits of change." Here, you are definitely *evoking*, the heart of good practice in MI (see Chapter 9).

● "I'm giving her time to envisage a plan that will work for her," or "I'm giving some advice and checking that it makes good sense to the patient." Here, you are *planning* (see Chapter 10).

Sometimes you can go through a consultation in a neat sequence, starting with engaging and ending with planning. Other times you need to move from one to the other in a less direct manner, perhaps going back to engaging at some point where things seem to go a bit astray. Either way, as long as you know why you are doing this, you'll be putting MI into practice.

You might find it useful to think of these processes as stair steps (see Figure III.1), starting with engaging and ascending through focusing and evoking up to planning, bearing in mind that you will often need to step back down to a lower step. Not every consultation will go in a neat order from engaging to planning, but the model at least provides a map of how you might proceed and why.

The next four chapters address each process in turn. Each chapter opens with some simple bullet points that summarize the main points of that process. Then we clarify what the process is and why it is important in the consultation. Then we turn to practical guidelines, like useful open questions you might ask, some examples of what the process looks like in practice, things you can try out yourself, and finally a few test-yourself questions.

After each of these four processes is described, the next part of the book brings them all together in various circumstances (see Part IV).

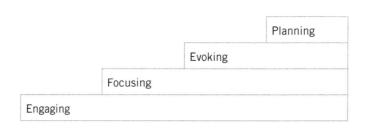

FIGURE III.1. Four processes in MI.

CHAPTER 7

Connecting with a Person
Engaging

I've learned that people will forget what you said,
people will forget what you did, but people will
never forget how you made them feel.
                              —MAYA ANGELOU

Engaging is more than being friendly.

Engaging happens when a patient feels that you understand what they
are experiencing.

MI offers a skill set for engaging, including rapidly in brief consultations.

The greater the challenge, the more useful engaging will be.

Engaging is essential for crossing boundaries of culture or language.

Engaging is often seen simply as being warm and friendly toward
patients. But, it is much more than that, and done well, engaging has
enormous healing potential. It is also a skill that can be practiced and
refined throughout your career. By engaging well, we mean adopting a
curious and compassionate mindset in which you use empathic listening to ensure the person you are talking to feels understood and empa-
thized with, throughout the consultation. MI rests on this foundation
of engagement. How to establish and maintain it is the focus of this
chapter.

Placing engaging at the center of care while also conducting so many other tasks is no easy matter. From a call like "Next please . . ." in a waiting room to a conversation driven by protocols and assessment, patients can begin to feel left behind and disconnected. Practitioners may feel overwhelmed by having to keep to their appointment schedule, not missing anything important, and making sure their records are up to date.

Our goal in this chapter is to make sure that, whatever barriers to engaging you may face, lack of skillfulness will not be one of them. Indeed, leaning on the skills described in Part II can make your professional life easier, not harder. We will illustrate how you can make every conversation count by starting well and reengaging whenever you feel the need to. Even with a patient you know well, there is considerable value in reengaging when you see them because even if their circumstances have not changed, their mood, expectations, and concerns probably have. Reengaging involves reconnecting about what really matters to them at that moment in time.

> **Skills like listening can make your professional life easier.**

Why Engage?

Engaging well brings benefits on multiple fronts. As you give patients an opportunity to say what they think and feel, you signal that you care about them as unique individuals, whatever their social or cultural background. They become more involved in treatment, and you get the opportunity to break free from the treadmill of seeing them as "just another patient" with this or that problem. For many practitioners, this single benefit—seeing patients as people first—is highly valued as an antidote to burnout and boredom because when you engage well, no consultation is ever the same as another.

A number of studies have highlighted that MI is helpful in crossing cultural and other potential boundaries in clinical practice. The emphasis in MI on engaging well is the most likely explanation. Indeed, the more complex and challenging the scenario, the more valuable engaging will be—for example, if a patient is feeling upset, angry, uninterested, or confused.

> **Seeing patients as people first is an antidote to burnout and boredom.**

Engaging also aids assessment and diagnosis because those little details you want to check up on often emerge in the course of a natural conversation. You can do two things at the same time: connect and assess.

> **CONSIDER: A Clinician's Voice**
>
> Being able to ask the right questions in an open-ended and nonjudgmental manner taught me to engage with patients on a deeper level than I thought possible in a time-limited setting. It showed me aspects of their lives that I never would have known if I had used the interrogative approach to interviewing that is common in clinical practice. It has deepened my empathy and resolve for wanting to practice medicine, and it has shifted the way I view myself and my interactions with others, both inside and outside of the hospital.
>
> —ANNIKA SHEARER, MD

The importance of engaging is well supported by research on empathy in practitioner–patient communication. Put simply, practitioners who are empathic tend to get better outcomes. The greater the cultural divide between patient and provider, the greater is the risk of dropout and the stronger the case for engaging in a sensitive manner (see Lee et al., 2019).

Engagement is often cut short by a practitioner interrupting the patient's opening account. While estimates vary, one recent study found that only a third of patients were able to outline their reasons for coming to see their doctors; when they were given room to describe their problems fully, it did not take them long, yet practitioners interrupted them an average of 11 seconds into the process (Singh Ospina et al., 2019). Under pressure of time and other forces, it's not always easy to avoid interrupting or diverting patients. The tendency to ask one question after another, without using listening skills, can interfere with engaging and leave patients feeling investigated and unheard, and *un*engaged.

Guidelines

It sounds simple enough to say, "Engage well with all your patients," but how do you do this?

Compassion and Curiosity

Compassion and curiosity are fundamental to good engagement—they allow you to focus not only on specific complaints and symptoms, but also on people's experience, their strengths, their community, cultural background and how they are feeling about the challenges they face. Your starting point is to find out about the person in front of you, or if it's in the middle of a consultation, to reconnect, however briefly, with how that person is feeling. In these moments, the aim is to be present and listen—and suspend other tasks, like asking diagnostic questions. With a mind free of such distractions, it becomes possible to harness curiosity to good effect. As you will see, this does not need to take a lot of time.

A Following Style

Using the following style described in Chapter 1, however briefly, is a discipline worth developing. When engaging with this style, you are an active participant not a passive recipient of the patient's story. You don't simply sit back and let the patient do all the talking. Here's an example from the start of a consultation, where the practitioner is fully engaged in listening, empathizing, guessing, and clarifying the patient's experience:

> PRACTITIONER: Please take a seat, you are looking a little flustered. [*Listening statement*] How can I help? [*Open question*]
>
> PATIENT: I am flustered because I am late for work, and I've lost all my energy. I don't know why I am so tired all the time.
>
> PRACTITIONER: You don't know what it is, but something's not right. [*Listening statement*]
>
> PATIENT: My daughter says I am overworking, but what can I do, we have to keep the house going. And then I have my own mother to think about. She is not well at all.
>
> PRACTITIONER: It must take strength to get up and make sure you get to work each day. [*Affirmation*]
>
> PATIENT: Yes, I guess so. It takes about all the strength I have got, to be honest.
>
> PRACTITIONER: And there must be times when you wonder how much longer you can carry on like this. [*Listening statement*]
>
> PATIENT: That's why I came down here. I mean I used to enjoy going to work, but now it's nearly impossible.
>
> PRACTITIONER: How were you hoping I can help? [*Open question*]
>
> PATIENT: My daughter says I am just run down, but I am not so sure.
>
> PRACTITIONER: And, you are hoping I can check you over to see what might be going on. [*Listening statement*]
>
> PATIENT: Yes, exactly, that's why I came down.
>
> PRACTITIONER: I'll examine you shortly, but before doing that, can

I ask you what you think might be going on here? [*Open question*]

Giving people space to tell their story cements engagement, particularly if you use listening statements to convey your understanding back to them. The more accurate you are, the sooner they may say something like "Exactly, that's right, that's how I feel." This allows you to move on efficiently, confident not only that you are on target clinically, but also that your empathic connection has been strengthened. Engaging in this way feels less like following *behind* the patient, more like walking alongside. Trust is developed with patients by your showing confidence in them **Engaging with a following style is like walking alongside the patient.** in the first instance. Doing that in a busy practice is not always easy, but certainly time-efficient and worthwhile.

A 20% Rule

Although engaging is important throughout the consultation, it is especially so in the opening phase. We developed something called the "20% rule" for engaging at the beginning of the consultation. More a rough guideline than a rule, the idea is to aim to use a following style and do *nothing but engage* for as much as 20% of the time available. As much as you might want to zero in on this or that topic, you hold back, like sitting on your hands, and resist the temptation to jump in with screening and evaluation questions, and only engage. We have found that any time apparently lost is made up for by speedy progress thereafter. Reports from colleagues seem to bear this out, particularly when the cultural background, presenting scenario, or diagnostic challenge looks like it could be complex.

Use Open Questions to Initiate Engagement

In time, as you become more proficient with the core skills presented back in Part II, you will notice a pattern emerging. As seen in that example above, open questions can be easily intermingled with listening statements and an affirmation, in what feels like a brief, free-flowing everyday conversation. Having a bank of useful open questions in mind can serve you well, either for starting things off or for reengaging at any time—see Table 7.1 for some suggestions.

A common concern about engaging and using a following style can be captured thus: "Ask an open question and they won't stop talking." If

TABLE 7.1. Sample Open Questions for Engaging

- "How are things going for you?"
- "How are you feeling day-to-day about your health?"
- "What matters the most to you today?"
- "How can I help?"
- "What's your understanding of . . . ?"
- "How did that come about?"
- "I wonder what you think is going on here?"
- "What's it been like these last few days and weeks?"
- "What concerns you the most at the moment?"
- "Tell me how you see it."
- "How do you want to use your good health in the years to come?"

you find a patient is running on in their narrative, consider the value of a summary (see Chapter 6), where you effectively take back control of the conversation by offering a summary that achieves two things: It allows you to make a transition to a new topic, and it ensures that the patient is onboard, because the summary confirms they have been understood. When people feel understood, they are usually happy to move on.

Engaging in Everyday Practice

We turn now to some common scenarios illustrating engaging in everyday practice. The first two are actually transcriptions of demonstrations developed for training purposes.

EXAMPLE 1: Brief Intervention; Emergency Room

The patient "John" wrote down on a screening questionnaire that he was homeless and using meth. He came in off the street, limping and looking dishevelled, with an injured wrist. Just a minute or so into the conversation, the practitioner decided to only engage for a minute or two. If you ask about a patient's everyday life first, it then is much easier to raise and explore a potentially tricky topic like illegal drug use.

PRACTITIONER: What is it like out there for you right now? [*Open question*]

JOHN: Tough, really tough. . . . I was in the army . . . got kicked out. . . . I don't like to talk about it . . . it's not a good thing. . . . I just struggle with that every day, got nowhere to stay. . . . It's so cold, it's always cold.

PRACTITIONER: So, there you were in the army, and you had some bad experiences you don't want to talk about . . . and you left the army and then it was like you landed in the streets. [*Listening statement*]

JOHN: I had nowhere to go . . . I was lost. . . . And I thought the only way to get through it, you know, meth. That's really f****** me up a bit to be honest with you, doctor.

PRACTITIONER: And, John, you have arm pain here (*pointing to his sore arm*), but what you are really saying is that soon after you came out of the army, there was a pain in your heart and your head. [*Listening statement*]

JOHN: Absolutely . . . a lot of mental health problems at the moment . . . and I've been struggling with it.

PRACTITIONER: A lot of pain in your mind, confusion. [*Listening statement*]

JOHN: Yeah, deep depression, not good thoughts, really dark.

PRACTITIONER: So, you felt really low when you came out of the army. [*Listening statement*]

JOHN: Nowhere to go, no one to talk to.

PRACTITIONER: And how did the meth help? [*Open question that initiates a focus on drug use*]

JOHN: It sent me away to another world, and I didn't have to be here.

It took less than 2 minutes, doing nothing but engaging, and it was then quite simple to establish the focus with an open question, "And how did the meth help?" The exchange started with an open question ("What is it like out there for you right now?"), and was followed by four listening statements, before that key open question about meth use. With a good connection and a clear focus on meth use, it was easy to move into the evoking process.

EXAMPLE 2: Outpatient Diabetes Consultation

In the above example, while the patient had plenty of troubles, he was not difficult to engage. The clinician just had to avoid getting in the way while John talked about his journey. It is not always so straightforward, of course. Here's another example, again a transcript from a training demonstration, but this time the conversation occurred with a patient who was quite angry. The practitioner used the core skills of asking and listening, and followed the 20% rule.

"Mr. Davies" was a patient with type 2 diabetes who had been coming to the clinic for many years, collecting his medicine and returning to his everyday life. He had a host of unhealthy habits that placed him at risk for health problems in the years to come. The practitioner in the clinic wanted to raise this issue with him, but got no further than 4 seconds into the discussion before Mr. Davies exploded with frustration.

PRACTITIONER: So, Mr. Davies, you understand you can continue taking your meds, yes?

MR. DAVIES: I got the meds. (*Raises his hand and stands up.*) I'm good.

PRACTITIONER: Mr. Davies, just one second, do you mind if you . . .

MR. DAVIES: Go on.

PRACTITIONER: Sorry, I appreciate that you're short of time . . .

MR. DAVIES: (*Interrupts, angry.*) No, you don't, I was waiting out there for half an hour. You set the appointment time on a day that isn't convenient to me (*Leans forward, pointing aggressively*) because it suits your clinic. Now I'm here, I'm on time, you're running late, now you've got to waste my time. . . .

PRACTITIONER: And you've made the effort to come down to the clinic today. [*Affirmation*]

MR. DAVIES: (*Interrupts.*) Yes, I certainly have.

PRACTITIONER: Which you do, I see from your records, you're a really good attender. [*Affirmation*]

MR. DAVIES: (*Interrupts.*) I'm a really good attender, I'm really good at taking my meds, that's all I need, let me go.

PRACTITIONER: I apologize we have kept you waiting.

MR. DAVIES: Oh, yes, because you can't run a system on time.

PRACTITIONER: You come in here wanting to be treated like an individual, and I guess you get to feel a little like you are on a conveyor belt. [*Listening statement*]

MR. DAVIES: I come in here because you summoned me. If I could just drop a note through the door and you give me a prescription, that would suit me just fine.

PRACTITIONER: So . . . whatever way you look at it, coming up to this clinic is not something you look forward to. [*Listening statement*]

MR. DAVIES: It's an interference. I manage all these things. You are just wasting my time.

PRACTITIONER: May I ask you to give me a few minutes just to chat with me this morning? [*Asking for permission*]

MR. DAVIES: I'm here now, let's get on with it. Say what you've got to say.

PRACTITIONER: Tell me how many years have you been coming up here. What's your story about your diabetes? [*Open question*]

MR. DAVIES: Look it up on the computer. You know, don't you? Actually, you don't know because you've not seen me before. There's always another bloody doctor.

PRACTITIONER: Exactly, that's right, I've worked in other clinics. I did look at your records, but to be honest, I didn't look at them carefully enough, and count the years. So, I just wanted to get a sense from you, what's it been like for you. [*Open question*]

MR. DAVIES: (*Calmer now*) What, coming here? Different doctor every time. There was one about 5 years ago, she was really nice, she listened to me. . . .

The rituals and procedures involved in the routine check-up can unfortunately strip people with long-term conditions of the essential human connection that drives quality care. Engaging helps to rectify this imbalance, and listening is a powerful way of defusing conflict, as was the case with Mr. Davies.

Listening is a powerful way of defusing conflict.

CONSIDER: When Engaging Is Really Tough

Some patients lie. They falsify their blood glucose records and forget their meters so you can't check. They know they are lying; I know they are lying, and they know that I know they are lying. Then what do you say? It's the kind of outpatient consultation that has me scratching my head wondering what to say next. They have the motivation to come to clinic but arrive with falsified glucose records so they can manage my expectations and be seen to obey instructions handed down to them countless times. So what do you say next? If you call them out, you risk them never returning. The service is somehow not meeting their needs.

—MOHIT KUMAR, MD

Engaging is all but essential if you are to overcome obstacles and prevent conflict, confusion, and poor outcomes. The dialogue with Mr. Davies is quite a dramatic example, and yet it captures the dilemma faced by many patients: Their treatment obliges them to undergo health checks and fails to engage them in a discussion about their needs. They become what might be called "professional patients," who know exactly how to navigate the system and get back home again. Engaging costs you nothing and, in cases like this, involves a commitment to connecting with people, and getting them involved in their health care. It is not an event, but a process, that over time usually leads to improvement in your work and the patient's well-being. One colleague put it this way: "I've often heard 'You mustn't trust them, they are lying.' But a client withholding the truth isn't breaking trust, it's being human. It isn't normal to divulge your private life to strangers. Build trust, and truth will follow. Don't expect truth before trust" (Shaun Shelly, personal communication).

EXAMPLE 3:   Reengaging in the Middle of a Consultation

Engagement fluctuates as you weave your way through the consultation, and sometimes you can unintentionally disturb it. Consider this example, not of skillful engagement but of the unintentional disruption of it:

> PATIENT: That's the story, thanks for asking. I've had this back pain for years now, and it gets me down to be honest.
>
> PRACTITIONER: How would you like best to get on top of this problem? [*Open question*]
>
> PATIENT: Well, I need these painkillers to keep going, not just at work. I can't sleep at night without them.
>
> PRACTITIONER: Are you aware that they are addictive? [*A closed question, unintentionally confrontational in nature*]
>
> PATIENT: (*Becomes agitated.*) Yeah, it's all very well for people in this clinic to say this and that, but it was here that they were prescribed. How else am I supposed to deal with the pain?

Here, the practitioner felt they had good engagement, so asked a simple question, and then the trusting connection took a nosedive. Under these circumstances, common in everyday practice, reengagement is a simple process that takes little extra time. You simply harness core skills to come back alongside the patient by doing a little listening for a while.

PRACTITIONER: My question gave you a bit of a shock. [*Listening statement*] My apologies. You feel like you did what was advised, and now it's not easy to hear a question about addiction. [*Listening statement*]

PATIENT: I heard the question. I just think it's a bit much to ask me about this now, 2 years down the line.

PRACTITIONER: This wasn't your fault, and you are still left with the back pain to deal with. [*Listening statement*]

PATIENT: Exactly right. Now we are saying I have two problems, not one.

PRACTITIONER: Somehow you want to find a way though this, but you are not sure how. [*Listening statement*]

PATIENT: Right again you are. I don't like living like this. [*Change talk*]

PRACTITIONER: It's hard to get on with your everyday life. [*Listening statement*]

Not only was reengaging brief and effective, but it is possible that the clinician's relationship with the patient was even strengthened as a result of the practitioner's "mistake."

EXAMPLE 4: Breaking Bad News

Imagine having to tell someone about a poor prognosis, or that because of deteriorating mental capacity (e.g., dementia), they can no longer drive a car. The skills involved are essentially those illustrated in earlier examples, where you engage throughout. Our experience with MI points to the value of getting into the right mindset, and staying in it.

- Instead of tightening up and rushing through the process, sit back and allow the conversation to unfold at a slower pace.
- Watch out for and resist the righting reflex, that temptation to solve the problem for the person, to offer premature reassurance, or to raise practical ideas to lessen the burden.
- Step down from the position of an authority on high to being more alongside the patient.
- Make use of a preparatory introduction, like "I know this will be difficult for you to hear. . . . " It can help to indicate that the situation is not unique to them and that you have had this kind of conversation with others.

Breaking bad news is a good opportunity to develop the skill of "sitting on your hands," being restrained as you deliver a simple message, practice empathic listening, and allow patients to ask those questions that make sense to them. How to handle change is in the hands of the patient, and your best position is alongside as a compassionate support. Here's an example where it is in the patient's best interest to stop driving. Notice the almost exclusive use of a following style:

PRACTITIONER: There's something I need to raise with you, and it might come as a bit of a surprise. With these very dizzy spells and double vision you are having, I am wondering about your driving a car. Until we get this properly diagnosed, I think it is best not to drive.

PATIENT: What? It is like my life will collapse.

PRACTITIONER: This comes as quite a shock this morning. [*Listening statement*]

PATIENT: Yes, they don't happen that often, so why tell me to stop driving?

PRACTITIONER: It is not easy for you to see why this is necessary. [*Listening statement*]

PATIENT: I can see that you want to work out why it is happening and that you want to be careful.

PRACTITIONER: Yes, there could be many causes of this dizziness.

PATIENT: Can't I just do my short trips to the supermarket?

PRACTITIONER: It is a risk you feel might be worth taking. [*Listening statement*]

PATIENT: Well, it is like you are taking my independence from me. (*Visibly upset*)

PRACTITIONER: This feels really tough. [*Listening statement*]

PATIENT: Very tough. I mean what if I can't ever drive again?

PRACTITIONER: It's not just the short term you are worried about, but how this might pan out more in the long term. [*Listening statement*]

PATIENT: I am just shocked now.

PRACTITIONER: You have been taken by surprise this morning. [*Listening statement*]

PATIENT: Completely, and what now?

PRACTITIONER: I need to do a few investigations, and ask you some more questions, and meanwhile I have a request for you.

PATIENT: What's that?

PRACTITIONER: Well, two requests really: come back and see me next week, and second, if you have a dizzy spell, please write down what happened before and after it, and how you were feeling, okay? We can then look at this together. I am going to see you through this, whatever happens.

PATIENT: Thank you, and I won't drive until I see you next week.

The use of a following style improved their relationship at a difficult moment for this patient. The place of MI in this exchange lies not just in the skills used (by no means unique to MI), but in the practitioner's awareness of what not to do. For example, she was restrained and held back from offering false reassurance, let alone using the righting reflex to suggest temporary solutions like taking a bus or taxi to do some shopping for the next week. Persuading someone out of discomfort will so often lead to a negative reaction. Quality engagement is healing in itself.

> **Quality engagement is healing.**

TRY THIS

1. **Useful questions.** Either during or after a consultation, consider your answers to the questions that follow. Indeed, if you have access to an audio recording of yourself in a consultation with a patient, you can then reflect about your engagement as a whole or locate moments where things were not quite right, where you might have done better to reengage more actively.

   - "How comfortable is this person in talking to me?"
   - "How supportive and helpful am I being?"
   - "Do I understand this person's perspective and concerns?"
   - "How comfortable am I feeling in this conversation?"
   - "Does this feel like a collaborative partnership?"

2. **Use an engagement scale.** What will happen if you openly discuss engagement with patients, and ask them what might help to improve your connection?[*] If you draw a line with a scale from 1 (low engagement) up to 10 (high engagement), and ask the person

---

[*]Thanks to Carl Ake Farbring, who first suggested this idea to us.

what number best captures "How well are you getting along?" or "How helpful is this discussion?", you are directly working on improving matters because the patient can tell you what will be really helpful.

This engagement scale can also be used more quietly as a guide you keep in your mind's eye as you speak with someone. Being aware of the quality of your connection can help you to make adjustments as you go along. The lower the score, the more you need to be modest and work on listening well to the person's views and experiences.

Another way to use this simple scale is when listening to a recording either on your own or with a small group of trusted colleagues. What number would you give to engagement level at different moments in the consultation? What is the best thing you did to improve engagement? Was it to stop asking questions? Was it to offer a really good reflection? Where did things go on a downward trajectory and why?

3. **Practice holding back.** How easy will it be for you to do nothing but engage at the start of a consultation? Our experience is that this takes practice. Consider the following steps to improve on holding back before jumping to diagnosis and treatment:

- Consciously choose a forthcoming consultation where you are going to try to break the habit of peppering the patient with closed questions.

- Before the patient comes in, take a few deep breaths and say to yourself something like "Hold it, stay back, let this patient tell their story." One colleague told us that whenever she wants to engage with a patient, she imagines herself sitting on her hands for a few minutes, a private signal to herself to hold back and not ask closed questions.

- Imagine putting on a different pair of glasses, ones that focus on strengths and the whole person, not their pathology or risk factors.

- Now ask an open question and use your skills to understand the patient's concerns for a short time. No investigative questions or diverting from the patient's story.

- Remind yourself of the value of a summary as you let go of control while the patient speaks. Eventually, you can use a summary to regain control and move the conversation in another direction.

4. **"What matters to you?"** Consider using "What matters to you?" as an opening question. Colleagues around the world explored and developed versions of this question into a system for both engaging and treatment planning that has transformed care in many settings (Zulman et al., 2020). The logic here is that from the outset of a meeting, you inquire about and respond to the patient's most important priorities.

Test Yourself

For each of the three scenarios below, what question or statement from you will be best for engaging the patient? Our answers appear below. (*Hint:* What will encourage the patient to talk freely?)

A. Someone walks into your office looking distracted and says, "I need help to stop work. I'm not well."

   1. "What sort of work do you do?"
   2. "What's the problem at work?"
   3. "Tell me what's been happening for you."

B. A patient says, "I need some advice from you about all these tablets I am taking for this heart thing. I get dizzy and I think it must be the tablets."

   1. "You are having these dizzy turns, and this has left you feeling unsettled and concerned about what's going on."
   2. "How soon after taking your tablets do you feel dizzy?"
   3. "Are you experiencing any other problems with your heart? Any pain?"

C. In the middle of a discussion about painkillers, a patient says, "It was you people that gave me these tablets and now you tell me I'm an addict."

   1. "This is not how you imagined it turning out when you first came for help."
   2. "I see in your notes that you were warned about the dangers here."
   3. "We can organize help for addiction if you would like this."

(Our suggested answers: A = 3; B = 1; C = 1.)

CHAPTER 8

Finding Direction
Focusing

If you don't know where you are going,
any road can take you there.
—LEWIS CARROLL

> Patients can be put off if practitioners make all the decisions about what to talk about or if they change the subject abruptly.
>
> Focusing skillfully with MI means ensuring that the patient is onboard when deciding what to talk about; often this concerns a change in patient behavior.
>
> Asking permission, laying out the options (if necessary), and respecting choice are fundamental to good practice.
>
> Agenda mapping is a strategy for choosing talk topics, including those that feel difficult to raise with the patient.
>
> Difficulties in the conversation can often be rectified by a return to focusing, to clarify that the patient is onboard.

If engaging means being connected to the patient, focusing refers to what change might be talked about during the consultation. The need for focusing usually arises as you set out in a consultation, but also at crossroads en route, or whenever a decision is made to shift direction. The word "signposting" is sometimes used to describe how a practitioner points to where the discussion will be going. By focusing in MI, we mean making this decision *together*.

Imagine you are speaking with a patient who is obese, and who is being treated for worryingly high blood pressure. He is a regular smoker and drinks alcohol most days. You decide to spend a few minutes talking about how he might lead a healthier life and prevent future problems. Where will you start? How do you decide what to focus on? And, how might the focus change as the conversation unfolds? Focusing can consist of a simple question asking permission to talk about something, or it might take a little longer to clarify the possibilities. Focusing means negotiating a meeting of your agenda for change and the patient's. How this is done skillfully, driven by compassion and a willingness to listen, is the subject of this chapter.

Why Focus?

Focusing involves bringing options into the open, either at the start of a conversation or even very briefly midway through it. Either way, you highlight the choices available that you could focus on. This not only provides structure to the discussion, but also, in turn, enhances engagement as a result.

Focusing allows you to spend your limited time on a change that you believe in and the patient feels will be most likely to improve their health. You spend less time on unproductive detours, and more time on a fluid journey through the consultation. After all, it makes little sense for you to focus on one route, for example stopping smoking, if the patient would prefer to start with getting more exercise. The point we reiterate throughout this book: People will make better progress if they harness their own motivation, rather than rely only on what you think is best.

Focusing means negotiating a meeting of your agenda and the patient's.

Here's another example: Imagine you are speaking with a patient with back pain, for which he wants another prescription for opiates. You are concerned about dependence on medication and have an idea that his getting more exercise would likely help with the pain. Deciding on the focus will be a challenge for both of you. Or, consider talking with someone who is feeling ill with a lung infection. You wonder whether it is the right time to raise the subject of smoking. And, how do you handle focusing when a patient raises their most pressing concern just as they reach for the door, after the consultation has apparently ended?

Focusing can be particularly useful if you want to raise a subject that is potentially difficult for patients to talk about because they might feel embarrassed, surprised, ashamed, or even angry if you raise it. The subjects of smoking, medication adherence, or alcohol and drug use when broached are common examples.

Guidelines

You can sharpen focusing in your conversations with patients in a number of ways. Key skills that help with focusing include stepping back for a broader perspective, reassuring the patient you will not impose your view on them, asking the patient's permission to shift focus, gently returning the conversation to the subject you're focusing on, and using an agenda-mapping strategy (see details on pages 82–84) to structure the conversation. As with any other process in MI, your use of core skills like open questions and listening statements is the driver of good practice. Many times when focusing, you step back for a short time and have a conversation about the conversation, to agree on the way ahead.

The Eagle and the Mouse

To navigate the consultation with skill, you have to be like both an eagle and a mouse. The mouse responds moment-to-moment to what the patient is saying, while the eagle keeps an eye on the big picture, what's going on and where you are heading next. It is the eagle who notices the need for focusing: "Can we just stop for a moment? We have been talking about your medication, and I want to make sure I also talk about your weight at some point if that's okay?" Or, "Could I now ask you to think about something different? What's going to help you get fitter and healthier over the coming weeks and months? How do you see this?" Adopting the mindset of an eagle is a valuable tool when you want to monitor and shift focus.

Have a conversation about the conversation, to agree on the way ahead.

Reassure: "There Will Be No Lecture!"

Patients often expect to be given a lecture about unhealthy behavior. They're likely not accustomed to receiving help from someone who is less an instructor, and more of a guide who involves them in decision making. Some patients are so used to being at the receiving end of expert instruction that they simply play out the role of a passive and obedient patient. Reassurance that you won't take on the role of an authoritarian can often produce a sigh of relief and prepare them for taking a more active role.

Ask Permission

Asking permission to talk about a change of some kind takes just a few seconds. If you sincerely champion the patient's choice not to go any further, it will enhance engagement and connection. Consider this simple transition from focusing into evoking:

> PRACTITIONER: How do you feel about us spending a few minutes talking about losing some weight? Or, would you prefer to leave this for today? [*Open question about focusing*]
>
> PATIENT: Okay, but I'm not sure, it might not be that easy for me to lose weight. [*Feeling ambivalent*]
>
> PRACTITIONER: It sounds like it might be a bit of a challenge for you. [*Reflection*]
>
> PATIENT: Yeah, it could be, I guess.
>
> PRACTITIONER: Before looking at how you might do this, can I ask you about the why of losing some weight? How do you see this helping you? [*Open question about evoking*]

Asking for permission helps you to steer the focus of the consultation in a transparent way, giving the patient a choice about whether to take this route. The more engaged you are beforehand, the more frank the patient will be with you. The last thing you want is for a patient to say, "Yes, okay," if they don't really like the idea. Using listening statements immediately after the question will reap rewards, not just for enhancing further engagement but to give the patient the freedom to express their motivation to change.

Permission asking can also be used some distance into the consultation if you sense that the focus is becoming blurred, when you choose a moment to step back and consider a change in focus, for example, "Can I just stop you here, and let us take a step back: Would you like to carry on talking about this, and search for a way forward, or would you like to talk about something else like. . . ."

> **Asking for permission helps you steer the focus of the conversation in a transparent way.**

Use Open Questions to Clarify Direction

A simple open question can cut through any confusion about the focus for change. Table 8.1 lists those questions we have found particularly useful when focusing. As you can imagine, the skill lies not just in the question you ask, but how you follow up on it with other core skills that encourage the patient to say what they feel about change.

TABLE 8.1. Sample Open Questions for Focusing

- "We could talk about changes in [a, b, or c], but what about you? What would be helpful for you?"
- "What change in your lifestyle would help you to take better control of your health?"
- "Are you happy to talk about your smoking, or would you prefer to leave this for another time?"
- "There might be some things you can do at home to look after your health. Would you be okay with talking about this?"
- "What feels most important to you? Working on your sleeping habits or getting more exercise?"
- "What sort of lifestyle changes make the most sense to you?"
- "Can we shift focus now? I wonder about spending a few minutes on your diet and exercise?"
- "You might think about some changes in your lifestyle. This could be a change in exercise or diet, or you might want to talk about your smoking. I am more than happy to share my views, but what about you?"

Avoid Changing the Subject Too Quickly

A common mistake, observed often in recordings of consultations, is when a practitioner settles on a change topic with a patient but then switches the focus suddenly, usually without signposting the shift to the patient, let alone checking with them about the wisdom of the shift. If the patient is feeling ambivalent about change, the message from MI is to give the patient a moment or two to see why or how they might resolve this uncertainty. Bouncing around from one topic to the next is not an efficient or helpful way to proceed.

A Mapping Strategy

We developed what we call an "agenda-mapping strategy" in the 1990s (Stott, Rollnick, Rees, & Pill, 1995) as a way of supporting people with long-standing diabetes to review their lifestyle and consider change. It turned out to be useful with other presenting problems and diagnoses. The agenda-mapping strategy takes the form of a map or list of potential changes the patient might like to consider making. This strategy enables us to take a step back and share views about the way ahead near the beginning of a consultation. We originally used the phrase "agenda setting" to describe this task, then adopted the idea of a map, because it more accurately reflects the unfolding nature of the consultation.

You can refine the mapping process into a few words. Or, you can expand it and produce a drawing with the patient, for example, by inserting words into spaces like those in Figure 8.1, each representing a different possible avenue for making improvements in their health.

Following these steps will ensure the focus is clear:

1. Ask permission to step back and consider the options for change.
2. Lay out the choices (e.g., diet, exercise, drug or alcohol use, medication). Consider the value of leaving one space blank for any other change the patient might like to introduce.
3. Ask the patient what change they might want to talk about and mention a topic you might like to address.
4. Decide with the patient what to start talking about.
5. Use the map during the consultation if you want to change focus and even keep it for use in later consultations.

You don't always need to go rigidly through those steps, and in time practitioners tend to find their own way of using agenda mapping to suit their own style and preferences, a bit like learning a new dance form. There's a blank circle in Figure 8.1. This represents any topic that the patient might like to raise. Highlighting this possibility can be useful when you want to widen the discussion beyond health behavior change.

Brief and creative adaptations of this mapping strategy include producing a colorful printed version of the map with possible talk topics that people can look at, even in the waiting room (Channon et al., 2007), or you can simply keep this map in your mind's eye as you verbally describe the choices open to the patient. Mapping is the principle of stepping back and encouraging the patient to agree on a focus that produces better outcomes.

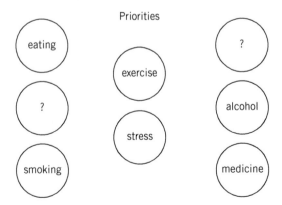

FIGURE 8.1. Sample agenda-setting sheet for use in a cardiac outpatient clinic.

> **CONSIDER: A Nautical Journey**
>
> I did my doctoral research on agenda mapping—how practitioners navigate their way through consultations that involve multiple possible directions for change, and a nautical metaphor turned out to be quite useful. In training workshops we thought of it like this: imagine making your way from one island to another, each representing a different possible topic for a change conversation; try to make decisions together about which island to go to, and then stay on that island until you reach a good moment to leave. Don't leave too quickly. Then signal to the patient that it's time to go and reach a joint decision about which island to travel to next.
>
> —NINA GOBAT, PhD

In summary, skillful focusing involves being aware of what you are talking about and why, and bringing patients onboard as much as pos-

Agenda mapping allows you to step back and share views with the patient about the way ahead.

sible, particularly in deciding about what change in health behavior they might attend to. It also involves not raising new topics without permission or in an unexpected way.

Focusing in Everyday Practice

Most times you can establish and maintain focus in an informal and naturally unfolding conversation by using the broad guidelines described above. The examples below all involve using the agenda-mapping strategy, not to imply that it should always be used, but merely to illustrate diversity of application. The other guidelines mentioned above are also addressed. With practice, you will develop your own way of helping patients address different change topics. The first two examples involve using pen and paper; the third example illustrates a less formal, purely verbal use of the strategy.

EXAMPLE 1: Routine Consultation, Breathing Difficulties

In this first example, the patient's presenting problem is difficulty with breathing. The topic arises in a routine clinic appointment. The practitioner is caught in the middle, wanting to practice with compassion and competence, yet aware that the patient needs to address issues in their lifestyle that are undermining their health. The patient in this example is approaching 60 years old, works part time, and has recovered some-what from a recent infection. She has been invited back to the clinic for a check-up. Her lung function is deteriorating, medicine can only do so much, and her smoking and sedentary lifestyle are clearly interfering with her recovery. She has four grown-up children and six grandchil-dren.

First up for the practitioner is to engage, with a person, not just a list of symptoms. It takes 3–4 minutes to discover the patient is a cheerful, friendly woman who is like a rock for others in her family, but someone with failing health. The clinician and patient clarify the plan for medical management, and the practitioner decides to focus on lifestyle using agenda mapping for the remaining few minutes of the consultation.

PRACTITIONER: You sound okay with the plan for medication, and yet you are heading back out there today to a very full life, with lots on your plate. [*Listening statement*]

PATIENT: That's me, for sure, and sometimes it feels like it's a moun-tain to climb.

PRACTITIONER: That's exactly what I am wondering, too. How you can keep your health and get to feel a little stronger?

PATIENT: No idea—I just take one step at a time, you know.

PRACTITIONER: Can we take a minute or two to look at your health and lifestyle, knowing that you will be the best judge of what is best for you. [*Introducing agenda mapping*]

PATIENT: Sure, okay.

PRACTITIONER: Here's a blank sheet of paper, and let's draw some circles on it, and fill into each one the kind of change you might make to improve your health.

PATIENT: I knew this was coming. (*Laughs.*) You will write "smok-ing" in there first.

PRACTITIONER: Well, I won't give you a lecture about this, but okay, can I write that word in here? [*Reassuring that there will be no lecture*]

PATIENT: You go ahead! (*Laughs nervously.*)

PRACTITIONER: Then what else? What comes to mind for you? [*Continuing with agenda mapping*]

PATIENT: Stress, too little time.

PRACTITIONER: So, stress goes in here in this circle for sure. And, could I place exercise in this circle?

PATIENT: Once again, go ahead. (*Smiles.*) Now that's a tough one because when do I fit that in? [*Sustain talk*]

PRACTITIONER: You can't see a way of doing it even though it might improve your breathing. [*Listening statement—a brief moment for evoking. Practitioner places the positive change part of the reflection at the end, like an invitation for the patient to talk about the value of exercise.*]

PATIENT: Oh, I've been told that many times here in the clinic, but it's not so easy. [*Sustain talk*]

PRACTITIONER: Whatever you do, you want to feel it is manageable. [*Listening statement; focusing attention on change, and what might work*]

PATIENT: Yes, that's right.

PRACTITIONER: What else might go into a circle? Diet?

PATIENT: Okay, put it down, I know I could be lighter with weight, but hey, who doesn't need to lose weight? [*Sustain talk*]

PRACTITIONER: So, we have quite a few areas in your life where you might just decide to think about a change that will keep you healthier, and here is a big question from my side coming up.

PATIENT: (*Interrupts.*) Here goes, stop smoking or else. (*Laughs.*)

PRACTITIONER: These are *your* choices. [*Emphasizing autonomy*] I wonder whether I can ask you to come back and see me personally in 2 weeks' time, so we can continue the conversation. I'll keep this drawing for us to look at next time. I can see it is not easy, but there might just be a change that you feel ready to make in any of these areas.

PATIENT: That's very kind of you, thank you. I promise I will think about it. [*Change talk*]

When there are multiple possible avenues for change, it usually makes sense to give priority to that change the patient is most ready to tackle. That's why the practitioner in Example 1 used agenda mapping to conduct a broad overview first, rather than diving into talking about any one behavior change, like smoking or exercise. The patient might prefer to talk about tackling stress. The consultation ended without agreement because the practitioner knew that with long-term conditions you have continuity of care at your disposal, and recognized it could be beneficial to sow the seeds for change, and then harness the patient's own good judgment when they next meet. One could debate whether this practitioner should have given a clear message about smoking to the patient before they parted. After all, what if the patient never comes for the follow-up visit? Sometimes giving the clear message about behavior change might work well; other times it can lead to the patient shutting down because the chances are a patient like the one above would have received the same advice beforehand. Sowing the seeds—setting an idea in motion—for change is a widely used strategy in health care.

EXAMPLE 2: Making Links with Agenda Mapping; Low Mood

Agenda mapping can be used to help a patient "see the forest from the trees," to make connections between different parts of their life so they can consider how best to make improvements. You don't focus in on any single problem or issue, but step back together and look at the links between them. Here's an example in a primary care consultation of a patient who is feeling depressed and has decided to seek help.

> PRACTITIONER: If we step back for a moment, can we take a wider look at your life and see where those low mood times fit in, and even what you do to lift your mood? [*Asking permission to use agenda mapping*]
>
> PATIENT: Okay, but I feel bad all the time these days.
>
> PRACTITIONER: It's hard for you to see any chinks of light, yet you don't mind taking a look at this with me. [*Listening statement*]
>
> PATIENT: No, but it feels a bit pointless most of the time.
>
> PRACTITIONER: (*Draws agenda map on paper with circles containing the words the patient and practitioner have come up with: low mood, eating, watching TV, exercise, going out of the house, diabetes, seeing a friend, etc.*) If we look at the big picture of your life at the moment, how do you see the links between these different parts of your life? [*Key open question*]
>
> PATIENT: It feels like a nothing life to me to be honest.
>
> PRACTITIONER: You don't feel good much of the time. [*Listening statement*]
>
> PATIENT: Yes, that's right. [*Sustain talk*]
>
> PRACTITIONER: But, what about the links, what do you notice? [*Returning to key question*]
>
> PATIENT: Oh, I see what you mean. When I feel depressed, I don't want to get any exercise, and then all I want to do is eat, watch TV. Is that what you mean?

PRACTITIONER: You can see a negative spiral there. [*Listening statement*]

PATIENT: Yes, it's there for sure. [*Change talk. The consultation moves naturally into the evoking process, guiding the patient to a new perspective about why and how she might break out of the spiral.*]

PRACTITIONER: You can see some habits that are not helpful. [*Listening statement*]

PATIENT: Well, that's why I came down to see you today, I feel stuck and don't like it. [*Change talk*]

PRACTITIONER: I wonder, if we look at the links here, what one small thing might break that negative spiral, somewhere to start at least?

PATIENT: I don't know, but sitting in front of the TV during the day does me no good. [*Change talk*]

PRACTITIONER: You're not happy about that little habit. [*Listening statement*]

PATIENT: No, it's not good. [*Change talk*]

Agenda mapping was used here to establish a focus for change that made sense to the patient. Also apparent was the way the conversation shifted between evoking and focusing quite naturally.

EXAMPLE 3: Raising a Difficult Subject

Raising a difficult subject can be a challenge, when you take a deep breath and wonder, "How will she react when I ask her about XYZ?" It might be alcohol use as in the example below, or it could be the theme of diet with a parent whose child is obese, or perhaps a concern about a patient's dependence on pain medication. In any case, we're often concerned that a direct or up-front approach to the topic might generate pushback or a shutdown. As we explored in Chapter 7, engage first, and it will be much easier to ask a difficult question.

The exchange below illustrates how agenda mapping can aid a smooth transition to talking about a sensitive topic, one the patient might feel fearful or reluctant to talk about. In this example, a man is sitting beside his bed recovering from an acute gastric episode that, from his medical records, is highly likely to be alcohol-related. A practitioner engages to begin with, and then turns to agenda mapping as a means of raising the subject. Hospital staff have described the patient as a quiet person, yet likely to react defensively. He holds down a job as a stock clerk in a factory nearby.

PRACTITIONER: So, you are feeling much better after what must seem like a scary time in the hospital, and you want to use all your strength to get back to work as soon as you can. [*Summarizing after 2–3 minutes of engaging*]

PATIENT: Yes, I think that's right.

PRACTITIONER: Would you mind if we talked about your health and daily life for a few minutes? Are you feeling well enough to do this now? I wanted to make sure we had a chat before you left the hospital. [*Asking permission*]

PATIENT: Yes, okay.

PRACTITIONER: How well were you feeling before you came into the hospital? [*Open question*]

PATIENT: Not too bad. I was working hard, and I never had too much time to think about this to be honest.

PRACTITIONER: I can see from your records that you live with your wife and that your son has now left home, yes?

PATIENT: That's right.

PRACTITIONER: If we look together now at your lifestyle, there's your job, your diet, your smoking—which I see is occasional— there's exercise, too. [*Introducing agenda mapping without pen and paper*]

PATIENT: Yeah, I don't smoke much and I don't get a lot of exercise, and my diet is okay because my wife and I eat regular meals and that sort of thing.

PRACTITIONER: Then there's alcohol. Where does that fit in for you? [*Raising the difficult subject*]

PATIENT: (*Somewhat defensive*) What, I don't drink all that much, maybe on the weekends more than during the week. [*Sustain talk*]

PRACTITIONER: Sometimes it is more than at other times. [*Listening statement*]

PATIENT: Yeah, on the weekends I like to watch sports and drink my beer, but I never get really drunk. [*Sustain talk*]

PRACTITIONER: Drinking is part of your everyday life. [*Listening statement*]

PATIENT: Yes, that's right.

PRACTITIONER: And this stomach problem, have you ever wondered whether there might be a connection with drinking? [*Closed question*]

PATIENT: Is that what you think?

PRACTITIONER: Well, maybe I could share some information with you and see what you make of it? [*Introducing the idea of information exchange using the ASK–OFFER–ASK strategy; see Chapter 11.*]

Agenda mapping in this example was used without pen and paper, as a way of establishing a focus by placing the delicate subject of alcohol use in a wider context of the patient's everyday life. The practitioner managed to raise the subject in a nonthreatening way as a foundation for evoking and helping the patient to clarify the links between his gastric symptoms and alcohol use.

TRY THIS

1. **Useful questions.** Simply having the distinction between engaging and focusing in your mind is a useful first step. "Are we well connected?" is a question about engaging, while "Are we talking about something that we both see as important?" is about focusing. If there is something not right in the consultation, it often calls for attention to one of these processes. When it comes to focusing, if you reflect on a consultation, perhaps by listening to an audio recording of it, do any of these questions strike you as relevant:

   - "Who decided what the focus would be, and to what extent was this a shared decision?"
   - "Did I have a clear sense of where we were going? And, what about the patient? Did they seem comfortable with the topic being discussed?"
   - "Did I change the subject abruptly?"
   - "What goals for change does this person really have?"
   - "Do I have different aspirations for change for this person?"

   You can start using the focusing map in Figure 8.1 with carefully selected patients when you feel engagement is positive, and there are clearly two or more choices about what changes they might consider. The strategy is not something done to or on a patient, but *with* them, and your style of open negotiation and willingness to hand over control to the patient is more important than the tool itself. You can also use this strategy in everyday life, for example, when uncertain about different possible decisions with a partner or young person. You might not need a map, but you can use words to step back from decisions and lay out the options with another person.

2. **Check your consultations: Who changed the subject, when, and why?** An audio-recorded consultation is a rich source of learning opportunities. If you stop at each point where the subject has changed, consider these questions:

- "Why did the subject change?"
- "What was the patient's reaction?"
- "If you changed the subject, was this based on good intuition or judgment, or with hindsight, would you have done it differently?"
- "Was the subject changed perhaps too quickly?"
- "Was the patient consulted? Might this have been a good idea?"

What happened to the level of engagement?

Test Yourself

For each of the three scenarios below, which best describes focusing with the patient? Our answers to each of these questions appear below.

A. Which of the following is an example of focusing in MI?

1. You ask a patient to tell you how they are feeling.
2. You inform a patient you will write a letter to a colleague on their behalf.
3. You ask a patient which area, exercise or diet, they feel most ready to talk about making a change in.

B. Which of these questions when posed by a practitioner is focusing with skill and compassion?

1. "I feel strongly that you should get a vaccine, and now is the time to tell you this."
2. "We are talking about you getting more exercise, but I wonder whether this is helpful to you right now?"

3. "Next on my list is your smoking. How do you feel about setting a quit date?"

C. A patient with asthma smokes occasionally and confesses that she often forgets to use her inhalers. Which of these practitioner statements is most consistent with focusing in the spirit of MI?

1. "My feeling is that you should focus on your smoking as your no. 1 target for better health."

2. "Your asthma is going to get worse over time if you don't use those inhalers properly."

3. "What feels most important for you to talk about today: your inhaler use or thinking about quitting smoking?"

(Our suggested answers: A = 3; B = 2; C = 3.)

CHAPTER 9

Addressing the Why and How of Change

Evoking

The most courageous act is still to think for yourself.
Aloud.
—Coco Chanel

> Persuading patients to change is fraught with difficulty.
>
> Evoking in MI means guiding people to give voice to their own good reasons to change.
>
> MI offers guidelines and skills for exploring ambivalence and for reinforcing the language of change used by patients.
>
> Evocative questions and strategies open up a helpful conversation about change.

Evoking involves helping a person to think aloud, and it happens at any point in the consultation when the focus is on a change for the better in the patient's life. It involves helping them to motivate themself, to come to a fresh perspective on what will be best. You guide them in a caring and compassionate manner, curious about how they might reach for that horizon, a healthier life.

Imagine you decide to explore someone's motivation to change, and that you are well aware of not jumping in with your own solutions or arguments for change. You ask a curious open question, and decide to simply let the patient say how they feel about change. You are now in the realm of evoking. This is how such a conversation might start:

PRACTITIONER: What might you do to improve your diet?

PATIENT: I don't know to be honest. Life is just so busy I hardly get time to think.

PRACTITIONER: If you had the time, you might be able to come up with a plan, but that's not so easy. [*Listening statement*]

PATIENT: Exactly, I want to do better than I am [*Change talk*], but I know it's hopeless to go on those diets. I just put all the weight back on again. [*Sustain talk*]

PRACTITIONER: If we take time now to think about this, what comes to mind?

PATIENT: I wonder sometimes about trying to . . . [*Change talk*]

Evoking is not complex and time consuming, and it does not mean sitting back passively while the patient does all the work, but rather using skills like asking and listening to steer the conversation to focus on why and how change might come about. Even offering information and advice can be brought into this activity, for example, by asking patients how they see the personal implications of the information you provide; that's when you will hear the change talk that indicates progress in MI (see Chapter 2). People hear themselves express their own good reasons to change. Feeling stuck is a common experience, and evoking is designed to help patients to break free from it, whether you are talking about why they might change or how they might achieve it.

> **Steer the conversation to focus on why and how change might come about.**

Why Evoke?

If you see each patient's life as a unique jigsaw puzzle, the case for evoking is a strong one; they are usually in the best position to know how the pieces might fit together. Evoking solutions from them is going to be more effective than imposing or dictating them. The more patients make their own case for change, the better their outcomes will be.

> **Evoking relieves you from feeling you need to solve the patient's problems for them.**

Another benefit to evoking is that it makes for a more satisfying experience inside the consultation. You can be relieved from the grip of the righting reflex, free from that feeling of needing to solve patients' problems for them.

Finally, evoking works particularly well when patients are ambivalent about change. This is not a comfortable state of mind to be in ("I can see that I should stop smoking, but it's my one source of stress relief at the moment"). Evoking helps patients to feel safe and brave enough to unlock themselves from the grip of ambivalence.

Guidelines

Evoking usually starts with an invitation to consider change, which often feels like you are stepping back and getting out of the way as patients talk about the possibility of change. What you bring is an attitude of curiosity and a keen eye on the change horizon.

Use Open Questions, the Answer to Which Is Change Talk

A simple clear route to evoking is to ask questions that elicit change talk. These questions provide the prompt for the patient to envision the road ahead. "How might you benefit from losing some weight?" is a good example. In reply, the person will hear themselves say out loud to someone, often for the first time, what this will mean for them, in the form of change talk. At this point, your best advice to yourself is not to rush ahead.

A useful tip is to imagine the answer to an evocative question *before you ask it*, to wonder about the patient's motivation and what kind of change talk might emerge.

> PATIENT: I thought you might ask me about losing weight. I just seem to be getting bigger and bigger.
>
> PRACTITIONER: (*Pauses a moment, imagining the answer to the question.*) How might you benefit from losing some weight?
>
> PATIENT: Well, to be honest, I want to . . . [*Change talk emerges.*]

Change talk varies in a number of ways, including in strength (see Chapter 2). There is a difference between "I really very much want to do this" and "It might be a good idea." Responding appropriately, without jumping too far ahead of the patient's willingness to change, lies at the heart of skillful practice.

Table 9.1 provides a sample list of open questions likely to evoke change talk. Open evocative questions like these can sometimes stick

TABLE 9.1. Open Questions to Evoke Change Talk

- "Why might you decide to make this change?"
- "What concerns do you have at the moment about feeling overweight?"
- "How do you see the benefits of _____ (e.g., quitting smoking)?"
- "What do you need good health for? What does it allow you to do?"
- "What ideas do you have for how you might decrease your alcohol use?"
- "What would you be willing to do to stay healthy as you age?"
- "What do you already know about the results of uncontrolled diabetes?"
- "What will it take for you to think about stopping smoking?"
- "How might you get to feel more in control of your health?"
- "In what way will taking your meds on time help you to get on top of this illness?"
- "How important is it for you to consider a change in . . . ?"
- "How confident are you about making a change in . . . ?"
- "How might you go about this to succeed?"

with people long after they leave the consulting room, even if they are not adequately answered within it.

Keep Steady When You Hear Sustain Talk

A common misunderstanding about MI is that it calls for the practitioner to ignore sustain talk in favor of a focus on change talk—that you don't want to give people time to talk about why they *don't* want to or *cannot* change. On the contrary, in your skillful conversations with patients, you need to pay close attention to sustain talk. It's a question of balance. Sustain talk is normal, common, and often simply one side of ambivalence. For example, you may hear it alongside change talk in a single utterance: "It might be good to lose weight (change talk), but I don't think I can do it (sustain talk)." While, of course, we don't want a focus on sustain talk to reinforce hopelessness, people frequently appreciate being heard. Listen to patients and reflect their sustain talk. When you do that, the relationship is strengthened and, as a result, it becomes easier to switch the focus to the positive.

CONSIDER: Sounding the Car Horn

We provide study days to help practitioners in sexual health improve their MI skills. Participants frequently report patients making confrontational statements that can feel threatening, like, "I'm sick of coming down here wasting my time," or, "I'm at the end of my tether trying to get guys to wear condoms." We have called this kind of client retort "Sounding the Car Horn," because it is a signal that change is often *just around the corner.* Stay calm, come alongside and give the patient space to express themselves. We now regularly include "Sounding the Car Horn" as a topic for discussion and practice in our study days.

—RICHARD WILLIAMS,
Society of Sexual Health Advisers, United Kingdom

Instead of backing away from it, skillful MI often involves reflecting back the sustain talk and then gently pointing the discussion in the direction of positive change. If the patient is clearly not ready for this, they will let you know. That is their choice after all.

Use Core Skills to Steer the Conversation

If the conversation is like sitting together in a sailboat, evoking involves keeping an eye on the direction of travel while giving the patient as much control of the steering as possible. In the consultation, core skills (open questions, affirmations, listening statements, summaries; see Chapters 3–6) allow you to gently support the steering so as to maximize progress for the patient. Using these skills also gives you time to notice, highlight, and gently guide the patient's attention to the positive case for change.

After asking an open question whereby you call for change talk, it is the use of listening statements that allows you to hear, reinforce, clarify, and support this change talk. The opportunity to use affirmation is present in most change conversations. Recall, affirmation helps patients to encourage themselves and be brave about making decisions to improve their health ("You have this determination and now you want to search for a way to take action").

When wrapping up the conversation, longer summaries have varied uses, but when evoking, they are like gold dust. You work through the conversation asking evocative open questions, which allows you to notice the change talk, the words and phrases patients use that indicate their strengths and motivation to change (e.g., "I want to . . ."; "I need to feel . . ."; "I think I should . . ."). If you log these words and phrases in the back of your mind as you go along, when it comes time to offer a longer summary, you can reintroduce these key words and the change, capturing and amplifying the essence of what the patient is feeling and thinking (see Chapter 6).

Sow the Seeds of Change

Patients often appreciate simply having the time to discuss a change even if they don't make a final decision to go ahead with it. As stated earlier, sowing the seeds for change often has an impact beyond the consultation.

CONSIDER: Speaking from Experience

I thought it was my responsibility that the patient agreed to change right there in the consultation with me. I would tell them what they needed to do and why and do my best to persuade and convince. Now I know that what is important is to create a space that allows them to open up and feel comfortable to talk to me without judgement. In this environment it is not about pushing a patient to change, rather to listen to their story with care and respect and ask about their ideas and thoughts about changing. If they are not ready, I summarize and then we end on a good note with encouragement from me to give this more thought and an invitation to come back and continue the conversation.

—JUDITH CARPENTER, *dietitian*

Many practitioners know the experience of treating a patient who comes back another time and says up front that they have changed as a result of an evocative question being asked, or an observation made, in an earlier discussion with you. Without knowing it at the time, you had sown the seeds of positive change with your questions.

> Imagine the answer to an evocative question before you ask it.

Evoking in Everyday Practice

The three examples below reflect different routes to the same end: inviting the person to say why and how they might change. The task of the practitioner is to capture what the patient is saying about change, particularly the change talk, and hand it back to them. Doing that provides the foundation for asking what steps they might take to improve their health.

If you are new to MI, the first example below is probably the best place to start, with a strategy we sometimes call "MI made simple." The scenario involves a patient who is fairly well motivated to change, but not free of uncertainty. The second and particularly the third example involve people who are much less ready to change.

EXAMPLE 1: MI Made Simple

The use of three evocative questions provides the framework for this strategy, which captures MI in an almost ideal form—efficient and purposeful, with talk about change driven by the patient.

> PRACTITIONER: Why might you decide to quit smoking? [*Evocative question 1*]
>
> PATIENT: It's becoming obvious now. My breathing is just too bad. [*Change talk*]
>
> PRACTITIONER: You're having trouble breathing. You can see something needs to change here. [*Listening statement*]
>
> PATIENT: Well, I can't carry on like this. I must do something. [*Change talk*]
>
> PRACTITIONER: How might you go about it? [*Evocative question 2*]
>
> PATIENT: That's the problem. I think I need something to help with withdrawal. [*Change talk*] Then again, that's just the first week or two, and then I'll get tempted again. Not sure, really.
>
> PRACTITIONER: You want plans in place that will work for you. [*Listening statement*]
>
> PATIENT: Yes, that's right.
>
> PRACTITIONER: So, what do you think you might do? [*Evocative question 3*]
>
> PATIENT: I think I should . . . [*Change talk*]

This patient was clearly quite motivated to change. Consultations won't be as straightforward in many cases, but keeping the framework in mind could give you a sense of direction about the ideal trajectory of a change conversation that is based on MI.

EXAMPLE 2: Ambivalence: The Importance and Confidence Strategy

This example illustrates the use of two key questions when talking about a change in behavior with a patient: "How *important* is the change to you?" (the *why* of change) and "How *confident* are you that you can succeed?" (the *how* of change). They can be used in brief conversations, as in the example below, or for a more in-depth exploration of ambivalence. Either way, the questions are like knocking on the door of motivation, and the idea is to use listening statements and affirmation while evoking change talk. Below, the subject is a change in the use of antidepressants for low mood.

> PRACTITIONER: Can I ask you, how important is it for you to use a new medication to help with your mood? [*Key question about importance*]
>
> PATIENT: I'm really scared of taking no medication and falling back into feeling bad [*Change talk*], but these old pills I've been taking are just terrible so some days, I just can't bear to take them, so I don't. [*Sustain talk*]
>
> PRACTITIONER: And now, you are hoping to find a new medication that might work better. [*Listening statement*]
>
> PATIENT: That's why I came down here today, I can't carry on like this. [*Change talk*]
>
> PRACTITIONER: You summoned the strength to come down and talk about what might work better for you. [*Affirmation*]
>
> PATIENT: My daughter said I should come down, and I said there was no point. Then I woke up one day and just called your office. [*Change talk*]
>
> PRACTITIONER: (*They discuss a new medication, and next the practitioner asks about confidence.*) How confident are you about taking these tablets regularly each day? [*Key question about confidence*]
>
> PATIENT: I know you say they only work properly if I take them regularly each day, I just hope I can do it. [*Change talk*] The thing is, when I feel bad for any reason, I just sort of give up and let things slide. [*Sustain talk*]
>
> PRACTITIONER: It's like you could lose control even though you don't want to miss doses. [*Listening statement*]
>
> PATIENT: Well, this time I could maybe try to . . . [*Change talk*]

When MI is working well, it looks and feels like a normal conversation, with two people on a journey facing in the same direction and working together to find a new path. The two questions about importance (why?) and confidence (how?) merely provide the scaffold for doing this. They can be supplemented by scaling questions, where the patients give you numerical ratings from 1 to 10 for importance and confidence. This allows you to elicit change talk by asking open questions about this rating.

Scaling Questions to Elicit Change Talk

When using a 1–10 scale for exploring importance and confidence, you can elicit change talk very easily. Imagine that the person gives you a number 6 for either importance or confidence. You can ask a question like "Why a 6 and not a 1?", and the answer will be change talk. Or, you can look higher up the scale and ask, "What would help to get this score up from a 6 to a 7 or 8?" and, again, the answer will be change talk.

The *why* and *how* of change can remain in your mind's eye as markers or signposts on the journey through the consultation. Simply asking yourself about the difference between why and how can help you to make skillful decisions about what to talk about. Whatever route you take, the idea is to provide the patient with the opportunity to envision change.

EXAMPLE 3: Strong Ambivalence

The ambivalence in Example 2 was mild and straightforward to address. Sometimes ambivalence carries more weight and feels more intense—such as when you raise the subject of alcohol with an elderly person who struggles to walk and you are worried about her all but secret drinking habit, or when you speak with someone increasingly dependent on pain medication, as in the example below. MI provides a style and skill set for doing no harm and opening up a discussion that has the potential to promote change.

It is 5 minutes into the consultation; this patient and doctor have met a few times before to address his lower back pain.

PRACTITIONER: Okay, I can see how much you are suffering with this back pain, and here are some of those meds again to take you through the period up to Christmas.

PATIENT: Thanks, I need those to be honest.

PRACTITIONER: Before you leave, can we chat briefly about the years to come and where you might be going with these painkillers for your back pain?

PATIENT: Why's that? Are you suggesting I stop using them because that's not in the cards. [*Sustain talk*]

PRACTITIONER: I am concerned about you becoming dependent on them, and yet for you, stopping this medicine doesn't feel like a good idea. [*Listening statement*]

PATIENT: That's right. It's not. [*Sustain talk*]

PRACTITIONER: It's hard for you to imagine a life without these meds. [*Listening statement*]

PATIENT: That's right, I need them, and they help a lot. [*Sustain talk*]

PRACTITIONER: If you look to the future, how are you hoping things will turn out for you with this back pain? [*Open question*]

PATIENT: Good question. I don't know. I feel more trapped in surviving each day so I can't answer that one.

PRACTITIONER: Being trapped in what? [*Open question to evoke change talk*]

PATIENT: I don't want to live like this, spending my time with back pain [*Change talk*], but the pills are all I've got at the moment. [*Sustain talk*]

PRACTITIONER: It is not how you would like things to turn out. [*Listening statement*]

PATIENT: No, but what can I do?

PRACTITIONER: I guess you would at least like a future where you can walk without pain. [*Listening statement*]

PATIENT: That's for certain. Simple things like walking without pain. [*Change talk*]

PRACTITIONER: Can I give you some information about these pain-killers, and then we can see what you think? [*The practitioner shares her concern about dependence on pain medication and how gradual reduction might be a way ahead. She also highlights how exercise strengthens muscles and makes it easier to walk without too much pain.*]

PRACTITIONER: That might be quite a lot for you to think about.

PATIENT: I never knew that, about how exercise might help to make my back stronger. [*Change talk*]

PRACTITIONER: It is something you might consider. [*Listening statement*]

PATIENT: Yes, I think so. I can start that idea of exercise. I think I can. [*Change talk*]

PRACTITIONER: Anything else strike you as useful? [*Open question*]

PATIENT: What you said about the painkillers is a worry [*Change talk*], but I'm no way ready to let go of them now. [*Sustain talk*]

PRACTITIONER: Perhaps we can discuss this next time I see you. From your side you hope to get going with some exercise. [*Listening statement*]

PATIENT: Yes, that's fine. One thing at a time.

Opening up a discussion on a solid foundation of engagement is sometimes as far as one can go when a patient feels very reluctant to consider change. There is every chance the man in the above scenario will think about this issue of dependence before the next consultation.

TRY THIS

1. **Useful questions.** Anytime you get to reflect about a consultation, or better still look inside one via a recording, there is an opportunity to consider some questions about evoking. Review a recent conversation you had with an ambivalent patient. Notice (or try to recall) when change was discussed:

   - "Was I curious, calm, and able to listen?"
   - "Where was the change talk and sustain talk in that conversation, and how did I respond?"
   - "What is the proportion of questions to listening statements?"
   - "How can I improve the quality and frequency of my use of listening statements and affirmation?"
   - "How well did I manage to avoid jumping in or cutting across when evoking?"

2. **Small-group exercises.** Trainers in MI have developed a range of simple exercises that allow you and your peers to enjoy getting better at evoking and responding to change talk (see also Rosengren, 2018). Paper and pencil can be used to construct and share useful evocative questions. Then you can take a step up in skill development—write down typical patient statements, whether they be change talk or sustain talk. One person reads out a patient statement, and the others then take turns to verbalize a response. Then move on to the next patient statement. Making the time to learn together over time in a regular peer support session has become an efficient way to boost skills in many health care teams.

3. **Practice evoking in everyday life.** There are times in everyday life when you are helping someone to learn something new, to address a complex challenge, or to make a decision, and you notice the righting reflex kicking in with a desire to simply tell them what to do. Being aware of this can help you to hold back and practice evoking instead, getting into the mindset of drawing out from a patient what they think is best. A good way to hold back the righting reflex is using an open evocative question instead, a skill that is easy to practice in everyday life.

Test Yourself

For each of the patient statements below, whether change talk or sustain talk, which reply is *most likely to steer the conversation positively toward talk about change*? (*Hint:* Imagine the patient's reply; answers appear below.)

A. "I need to think about making a decision about losing some weight."

   1. "But, you are not sure it's the right time."
   2. "Why would you want to do that?"
   3. "I agree. It will help a lot with your health."

B. "I'm not sure. I could stop smoking if I wanted to, but why bother now?"

   1. "You would benefit a lot by making a decision to quit."
   2. "You feel it might be too late to try."
   3. "It is something you might consider at some point."

C. "It's a good idea to change my diet, but I can't do that at the moment. It just won't work for me."

   1. "Why's that?"
   2. "What will help you the most to succeed?"
   3. "What about simply taking one small step that is easy to adjust to? Then at least you are making some progress."

(Our suggested answers: A = 2; B = 3; C = 2.)

CHAPTER 10

Heading Into Action
Planning

A goal without a plan is just a wish.
　　—ANTOINE DE SAINT-EXUPÉRY

> Most of the wisdom about what will work best is inside the patient.
>
> Jumping ahead of patients' readiness is unhelpful, as is using the righting reflex to solve challenges for them.
>
> A *jointly* constructed plan for change is an ideal scenario.
>
> MI provides guidelines and skills for evoking a plan from patients and for sharing your expertise with them.

Planning happens when the patient seems ready to consider taking action. This does not mean they always *will* make a plan, let alone act on it, but it does signal the value of getting as far down the road to a change plan as possible. Some people walk out of the consulting room with a half-formed idea and then surprise you by making substantial changes. Less pressure and urgency from your side usually make for better outcomes, even in difficult circumstances for the patient. *How* you plan with a patient is just as important as the ideas you both come up with. In this chapter, we share the best of our experience of doing this in an MI-consistent manner.

Consider this exchange:

PATIENT: My daughter is pregnant now, and here I am gasping for breath with this lung problem.

PRACTITIONER: You would like to be as fit as possible for the birth of your grandchild. [*Listening statement*]

PATIENT: Yes, definitely, not just for the birth but as they grow up, too. [*Change talk*]

PRACTITIONER: What might you do to give yourself the best chance? [*Open question about change*]

PATIENT: It's got to be getting more exercise, and maybe I will also lose some weight. [*Change talk*]

PRACTITIONER: You feel quite determined to do something. [*Affirmation*]

PATIENT: Oh, yes. I can be strong when I want to get something done. [*Change talk*]

PRACTITIONER: How might you exercise more? [*Open question*]

PATIENT: Well, not at night because it's not safe out there. [*Sustain talk*]

PRACTITIONER: Something during the day. [*Reflection*] Is there anything I can help or advise you about?

When using MI to make plans, you will notice two things happen: Patients are motivating themselves, rather than just relying on you, and they are developing clarity about what they will do, how and when. Throughout this activity, you are *evoking* a clearer vision of what might be, noticing the strength of change talk, responding with care, asking what a good plan will look like, and offering your ideas and advice as needed.

How do the four processes work when planning? They are all firing when planning is going well: You are helping the patient to feel comfortable (engage), talking about a specific change (focus) while you elicit their best ideas (evoke) about what might lead to lasting change (plan).

> Notice patients motivating themselves and developing clarity about what they will do, and when.

Why Use MI When Planning?

Planning to make changes happens naturally, for better and worse, yet in the presence of a caring practitioner, people often make some remarkable decisions and then act on them. A conversation with a patient about change can also be frustrating, for example, when you feel on the cusp of making excellent progress with a patient, then get frustrated when your best advice seems to fall on deaf ears. There are few scenarios that call more strongly for using MI than conversations about planning. A decision to change and a plan that follows is a privilege to witness. In one study of brief MI, Lee and colleagues (2010) approached heavy drinkers in an emergency room and found that completion of a change plan predicted less drinking a year later. Planning skillfully changes lives.

Your attitude, reflected in your approach to planning, is key here. MI helps to steer you away from an approach in which the patient is seen as some kind of blank canvas, ready to absorb all your wisdom about what to do. Experience would soon tell you otherwise, when they react against the use of the righting reflex. MI offers the simple idea that we have returned to a number of times: It is best not to see yourself as a rectifier of what's wrong, urging and cajoling the patient to get a grip on their resolve and make this or that change. Instead, eliciting their own motivation and good ideas makes for a more satisfying and effective consultation. The aim is to do this efficiently, supported by your best advice.

Few scenarios call for using MI more than conversations about planning.

Guidelines

How you conduct the conversation about planning is as important as what you talk about, whether you use the "Why, What, and How" framework or one like SMART (Doran, 1981), both illustrated below. To succeed when using MI, the idea is to view the patient as a person with strengths and wisdom, to encourage choice, and to *offer* your best advice, not impose it. The skillful MI practitioner will hear and acknowledge talk about why things might be difficult (sustain talk) and still be able to steer the conversation toward what might work (change talk).

Clarify Readiness

Sometimes it is obvious when someone is ready to make a plan, but if not, a good place to start is to clarify with them just how ready they are. A common mistake is to assume greater readiness than is the case—you experience discord, the route out of which is to reengage and make a decision about whether to continue with planning. "How ready do you feel to make a plan?" is an example of a useful open question. Another is, "Would it be helpful to talk about a concrete plan, or is now not the right time?"

With MI you can acknowledge why change might be difficult yet still steer the conversation toward what might work.

A Readiness Scale

Some practitioners take advantage of the idea of readiness to draw a line and ask the person to say where they are on it, or to provide a number from 1 to 10, for example, by asking, "On a scale from 1 to 10, how ready do you feel to make a plan to lose weight?" If a patient offers you a number like 7, two further questions can be helpful: "Why a 7 and not a 1?" and "What would help for your number to go up from 7 to 8 or 9?" In both cases, the answers take the form of change talk, the driver of motivation. With the second question, you also get clues to what will really make a plan succeed.

Clarify What the Person Needs

"*What will be most helpful?*" A simple question of this kind, which hands control of planning over to the patient, can be quite helpful. People are so different. Some know what they need to do and will simply benefit from making a commitment in your presence. Others are unclear or feeling overwhelmed about the journey ahead and need help to work it out in greater detail. This is when you need curiosity above all else, along with an ability to grasp where the challenge lies and feed this back to the patient. The Why, What, and How framework presented below provides a rough guide to where the patient might need the most help. What's usually needed here is not cleverness on your part, but faith in the benefit of a joint search for possible solutions.

Why, What, and How?

Thinking about the difference between "Why?", "What?", and "How?" can provide a useful steer through the planning process (see Egan, 2013; Sinek, 2011). Using MI allows you to navigate this terrain with the patient center stage as you move between the questions to bring the plan into sharper focus. Here's an example, a continuation of the exchange started in Chapter 9, about the woman with breathing difficulties:

> PATIENT: Those streets are dangerous for an old woman like me panting along trying to get my breath. I'm an easy catch for those young hooligans.
>
> PRACTITIONER: That won't work for you, yet you seem determined to find a way to get more exercise. [*Affirmation—addressing the "Why?"*]
>
> PATIENT: Yes, because it's me that counts now, to get as healthy as I can. [*Change talk*]

PRACTITIONER: What might work for you? [*Addressing the "What?"*]

PATIENT: I could at least walk up the stairs in our apartment each day. [*Change talk, about both "What?" and "How?"*]

PRACTITIONER: You are beginning to see a plan. [*Reflection*]

PATIENT: Maybe that could work [*Change talk*], but when I get breathless, I sometimes need to sit down and I can't do that on the stairs. [*Sustain talk*]

PRACTITIONER: So, that's a problem you want to solve somehow. [*Reflection*]

PATIENT: Maybe I could . . . [*Change talk*]

PRACTITIONER: May I give you some advice?

Why?

Asking about and clarifying the "Why?" is worth its weight in gold. Ambivalence and uncertainty will undoubtedly ebb and flow as people move forward, and eliciting the "Why?" helps to fuel their motivation to keep going. Only occasionally do people have a moment of insight and make a quantum leap into change, free of doubt.

"Harnessing the heart" is one way of putting it, when you use those questions, reflections, and affirmations that help patients express their commitment to change. One example above was the affirmation, "You seem determined to find a way to get more exercise." The reply was full of commitment: "Yes, because it's me that counts now, to get as healthy as I can."

When planning, it is easy to focus on behavior change, but behind behavior sits the heart, patients' values, and motivation to make a success of things. The examples that follow illustrate how you evoke answers to the "Why?" question as an integral part of the planning process.

What and How?

Effective planning involves developing clarity and purpose about exactly what change stands the best chance of success, and specificity about how this will come about, when, and with what ongoing support. Some patients can see what's needed quite quickly, others need more time. Some appreciate the offer of advice and brainstorming, others less so. It is usually a good idea to start broad and general, and then narrow things down as the conversation unfolds.

Frameworks like the SMART model can be useful to clarify what you are looking for: a plan that is Specific, Measurable, Achievable, Relevant, and Timed (Doran, 1981). Many elements of this model are apparent in the dialogue above. Sharing this model with the patient can sometimes prompt useful reflection. What MI points to is that *how* you elicit a plan using a SMART model is as important as its content.

What's needed is not cleverness but faith in a joint search for solutions.

Open Questions to Firm Up a Plan

Table 10.1 contains a sample of open questions about the "What?" and "How?" of change. As in any other kind of change conversation, questions merely open the door. Listening statements and other core skills will be framed around action as you guide the person to imagine a workable plan (see Resnicow, McMaster, & Rollnick, 2012).

Imagining Together

Much of the power in MI involves the patient imagining how things might be different. Consider the difference between "What are you

---

TABLE 10.1. Useful Open Questions for Planning

- "What is it in this plan that's going to make the biggest difference to you?"
- "What will be most helpful?"
- "Of all the ideas, what feels best to you?"
- "What's your next step?"
- "What might work the best?"
- "How would you know when you are succeeding?"
- "How exactly do you see yourself succeeding with this plan?"
- "What feels the most manageable?"
- "How many ways are there for you to do this?"
- "How would this work out ideally for you?"
- "What would be happening?"
- "What will you do first? When?"
- "What would you be doing to succeed?"
- "What might you have overlooked?"
- "When do you want to do this exactly?"
- "How can we keep in touch to support you best?"

going to do?" and "What *might* you do?" With the second question, the patient will feel less pressure and more freedom to paint a picture of what a workable plan might be. A marker of skill when planning is the use of language that takes pressure off patients and gives them just a little time to wonder what might work.

Providing Quality Advice

It is during planning that information and advice can transform the consultation, for either better or worse. What makes a real difference is not only the content you choose to share but also when and how you do this. Chapter 11 provides a framework and examples of what worked well when it comes to advice giving. Using MI involves avoiding the mistake of assuming that the patient is 100% ready to change and wanting to absorb your advice; instead, you never let go of the principle that much of the wisdom is inside the patient. They will know where your best information advice will fit into their daily lives.

Change Plans, Diaries, and Monitoring Progress

An ideal scenario for many practitioners is a patient who completes a detailed change plan, along with a commitment to monitor their progress and report back. Skilled practice when planning with MI involves keeping an eye on the value of these activities without imposing them on patients. Not everyone wants or needs to do this in order to succeed. However, a simple open question can evoke commitment and a willingness to make the change happen, for example, "How will you monitor progress?"; "How will you keep on track?"; or "How useful will it be to make a detailed plan and even keep a diary of some kind?" The answers will depend on the person and the setting. Practitioners in remote rural settings might use text messages to keep in touch, while those working in the diabetes field, for example, will have access to sophisticated apps that monitor and share relevant medical data.

Planning In Everyday Practice

Illustrated in the scenarios below is how planning can be done using MI at its center, where all four processes are active, the language of change is attended to, advice is offered as needed, and plans are made with a sense of shared purpose.

EXAMPLE 1: Starting Broad, Getting Specific

This example spans a number of consultations, and has relevance beyond the specific setting, a clinic for young people with type 1 diabetes. The practitioner places high priority on not just being friendly, but being curious, and using the technical skills of open questions and reflection to help the young person feel connected and understood, and to evoke from them what a good plan for cutting out beer drinking might look like.

> PRACTITIONER: What would be the best for you now looking ahead?
>
> PATIENT: Don't know, really.
>
> PRACTITIONER: You want to get healthier, but you are not sure where to start. [*Listening statement*]
>
> PATIENT: Yeah, I don't know.
>
> PRACTITIONER: You are feeling down about things and want to feel better. [*Listening statement, a guess*]
>
> PATIENT: Yeah, I sort of hate this diabetes.
>
> PRACTITIONER: Your friends don't have it, and this feels unfair. [*Listening statement*]
>
> PATIENT: Yeah.
>
> PRACTITIONER: You've managed to keep going with your monitoring.
>
> PATIENT: Yeah, I have, and I want to lead a more normal life. [*Change talk*]

At the next meeting, the young man is feeling more connected to the idea of getting help. After asking him how he felt about coming down to the clinic, the practitioner continues:

> PRACTITIONER: If there was one challenge you feel ready to face, what might it be? [*Open question about the "What?"*]
>
> PATIENT: I want to stop the beer thing when we are at parties because it shoots my sugar levels through the roof. [*Change talk*]
>
> PRACTITIONER: You want to stop that happening and to also feel like you can enjoy yourself. [*Listening statement*]
>
> PATIENT: Yeah.
>
> PRACTITIONER: You feel that you have the strength inside you to go for it. [*Affirmation*]
>
> PATIENT: Yeah, I must. [*Change talk*]
>
> PRACTITIONER: So, what might a good plan look like, for keeping

your sugar levels down at a party and cutting out the beer? [*Asking about the "How?"*]

PATIENT: Don't know.

PRACTITIONER: What if I go through two or three ideas, just possibilities, and perhaps one of these might work for you, or they might trigger an idea of your own? [*Offering ideas about "How?"*]

PATIENT: Yeah, okay.

[*The practitioner presents three ideas: drinking a nonalcoholic beer; drinking a diet soft drink instead of beer; and asking a friend to drink whatever he drinks, a soft drink or a nonalcoholic beer.*]

PATIENT: My mate Jack would help me if I asked him, to drink a nonalcohol beer as well with me. [*Change talk*]

PRACTITIONER: That might work well for you. [*Reflection*]

PATIENT: Yeah.

PRACTITIONER: Tell me how this will actually work out for you.

PATIENT: How do you mean?

PRACTITIONER: Like what will you say to Jack?

PATIENT: Oh, Jack, he knows about my diabetes, so I will tell him why I want to leave out the beer. Then I will ask him to drink what I drink just for company.

PRACTITIONER: And if you don't mind my asking, when will you do this asking?

PATIENT: When I next see him, maybe later today.

PRACTITIONER: So, you have a plan here that's coming together. When is the next party?

PATIENT: Weekend probably.

[*They make an agreement for the patient to send a text message to the practitioner before and after the party.*]

There are two reasons why MI might be particularly powerful when planning: First, you have access to the skills for building a supportive relationship and, second, you have guidelines for evoking as much of the plan as possible from the patient.

EXAMPLE 2: Premature Planning

Sometimes you and the patient get sucked into planning talk prematurely, and you will most often notice this in the form of sustain talk of some kind, for example, "Yeah, that might be a good idea, don't know really." Another more subtle expression of a patient not being ready is what could be called "hollow change talk" where it all sounds a bit too good to be true, like the person is telling you (or themselves) what they think you want to hear, but it lacks conviction. You'll notice this in the opening statement from the patient in this exchange:

> PATIENT: Yes, I think I'll speak to my partner and we can make a plan together, and then it is more likely to work I guess, and then if we can buy food together, we can cook without frying too much, so thanks for the advice. I can see a plan here, and I also know that there are foods out there that will make a difference if you see what I mean, and also . . .
>
> PRACTITIONER: Can I stop you for a moment, if that's okay? (*Patient nods*.) Can I ask you a simple question: Why do you want to do this?
>
> PATIENT: Sorry, I don't get you.
>
> PRACTITIONER: In what way do you hope to really benefit from this change? [*Restating the "Why?" question*]
>
> PATIENT: Me? Well, of course, I want to change.
>
> PRACTITIONER: Why?
>
> PATIENT: Oh, I see now. You want me to think about this (*Speaking more slowly and looking more engaged*). I don't know. I can't carry on with just gaining more weight and my partner looks at me, and thinking I am getting ugly. [*Change talk*]
>
> PRACTITIONER: You want to feel better about yourself. [*Reflection*]
>
> PATIENT: I am tired, to be honest, of stuffing myself with junk food (*Becoming tearful*).

When you notice what feels like premature planning and hollow change talk, consider stepping back from the conversation with the patient, whether this is while you are evoking or planning.

CONSIDER: Taking a Step Back

We knew each other well, and he was up against many challenges with his health, addiction, poverty, and access to his children. He was a proud man in his forties, and as the change talk came tripping off his tongue ("I'm going to . . ."; "I must now . . ."; "Yes, I will walk out of here and . . ."), I started feeling that this was hollow change talk, that it lacked conviction. And I was confused about whether he was trying to make me happy or perhaps persuade himself about the strength of his conviction. Instead of trying to fathom it out, I asked him to stop for a moment and inquired: "Can I ask each of us to say how we are feeling right now?" "You first," he said playfully. I insisted he go first, and his answer was: "I'm feeling very scared." So we stepped away from planning and returned to evoking, with a stronger connection, and a more useful conversation unfolded.

—STEPHEN ROLLNICK

Test Yourself

For each of the patient statements below, which reply from you is most likely to help them feel understood and comfortable during the planning process? (*Hint:* Imagine the patient's reply; answers appear below.)

A. "I don't think that will work. I just don't have the willpower."

1. "How about trying just once, and then you can prove to yourself that you can?"

2. "Okay, so let's try this." (*Suggesting something else*)

3. "You are trying to find a way, and this idea might not be the best."

B. "How do I avoid the withdrawal symptoms of smoking?"

1. "You will want to make a plan that involves lots of exercise, new routines, and that sort of thing."

2. "There are some medications you might try, or were you thinking of something else? What makes sense to you?"

3. "You can't really—there's no gain without pain."

(Our suggested answers: A = 3; B = 2.)

EVERYDAY CHALLENGES

Here are 20 health concerns we picked out at random from a list of over 1,500 controlled trials of MI (we could have chosen 50 without difficulty). Take a look at this list, and consider what links them: diabetes, depression, cocaine use, child maltreatment, multiple sclerosis, diet, hemodialysis, being overweight, familial cancer risk, tooth decay, chronic kidney disease, medication adherence, HIV/AIDS, vaccine hesitancy, rehabilitation, cardiovascular disease, smoking, physical activity, enuresis, and suicide prevention.

At first glance, the diversity is staggering, but a common thread emerges: Patients with these problems are all facing the need to make adjustments in their behavior. They might be suffering with a range of conditions, living in very different circumstances and cultures, but whatever the problem, MI has been viewed as a broad framework that enables a constructive conversation about change to take place.

So, what is it about MI that is helpful across such a wide range of conditions and problems? It is not or should not be because practitioners are using MI to "chase down" behavior change at all costs, but because they are focused on connecting with people who have the wisdom within to know what's best for them. Our friend and colleague Shaun Shelly puts it this way: "If you sit in front of a patient, and you are 100% present, you listen and hear them without judgement or pity, and you encourage them, you can offer them a temporary scaffolding on which to hang an image of their future self, until they believe they are worth it and grow and learn to become the change they want. You will throw theory and labels out of the window and work according to their needs." Using MI, you arrange the conversation so that the patient feels connected, focused on improvement, and willing to say what this will look and feel like.

It is upon this foundation that we wrote the chapters in Part IV. Each has a particular focus, and all are united by a set of principles we spelled out in Chapter 1: you view them as people first, patients second; you place high value on connecting well; you work with their strengths, not only their problems or deficits; you champion choice and believe they are capable of making wise decisions about their lives; and if applicable, you *offer* advice rather than impose it.

CHAPTER 11

Offering Advice and Information

When a client asks me for my opinion, I don't avoid giving it.
I simply say that first I want to hear what they think because
I believe they may already have a big portion of the answer
within them, and after that I will add my own thoughts.
—TONU JURJEN

Imagine you are a mentor and friend to a practitioner who flies out to a remote African village where there is an outbreak of smallpox, which had been unheard of until this moment. This terrible disease, which killed over 500 million people, mostly children, was thought to have been completely eradicated many years back. Now there is this outbreak. Your friend's job is to give vaccines to all in the village, and this young father she meets says he doesn't want to take it. What now? How should your friend proceed? Persuasion is unlikely to work well. How might she offer information and advice in a helpful way that makes a difference?

This chapter outlines and illustrates a framework for giving information and advice that not only works well in tough circumstances but can also be blended with MI. These messages can inspire and change lives if delivered with skill and compassion, or land with a dull thud if presented as cold dictates. This chapter clarifies the difference and illustrates the integration of advice giving with MI. Get it right and it feels satisfying, impactful, and even artistic.

Giving information and advice can be blended with MI.

With its emphasis on passing on messages *to* the patient, giving advice might at first sight seem incompatible with MI, which relies so much on drawing ideas and inspiration *from* them. Can these two

119

apparently contrasting approaches, providing and eliciting, be reconciled and integrated? We believe they can if you focus particularly on *how* you give advice, not just what the content might be. The key is to *offer* rather than dispense advice and listen to what sense patients make of it.

Practitioners often complain that patients don't listen to their advice, and data on poor levels of medication adherence and other suggested changes would seem to back this up, with life-threatening consequences so often there for all to see. What we are suggesting is a two-way process. If you listen more to patients, they will listen more to you.

Offer advice, rather than dispense it.

Before looking at the practicalities of giving advice, pause for a moment to consider it from the other side, the experience of patients. What happens when a patient is feeling confused, anxious, or distracted and the practitioner dives straight in with information or advice, without engaging first and giving them a moment to absorb, reflect, or ask questions?

CONSIDER: A Patient Has Zoned Out

"How many times must they tell you?" It was my loyal and very concerned son speaking, getting frustrated about how little I understood about why I had had this heart attack, even though, as he put it, "They told you once, they told you twice, and you still don't get it. What's the matter with you?" From my side, I mumbled and fumbled in reply, and looking back now, I think I can see the problem. The doctors were good people, and they delivered the information a bit fast, but I just wasn't receptive. It was a routine low demand scenario for them, but a high demand one for me. I was zoned out.

—STEPHEN ROLLNICK

Getting It Right

There are a few ideas and practices that can help you give advice and information effectively. Keep in mind, first of all, that this is not the only tool in the toolbox. In fact, think of it as something to be used judiciously and only at the right moment. You want to avoid using it in the service of the righting reflex (see Chapter 1), trying to solve every problem in front of you.

Second, view advice giving as an offering, a two-way process, one that includes not just your contribution but also an opportunity for patients to say what they want, need, and can use. You impart knowledge and ideas, but you also ask patients questions and listen to their views and aspirations.

Third, be mindful of the psychology involved. People tend to back off from unwelcome messages, quite understandably, and they like to have autonomy in making decisions, particularly those about their own health. It's common for a patient to feel ambivalent or uncertain, which means it's best to approach them without pressuring them.

The language you use can be particularly important when empowering people to consider your advice. "One thing you *should* do . . ." will land differently than "One thing you could consider doing. . . ." Advice giving reaches a high point in skillfulness when your language is fine-tuned. "Offering" advice is quite different from delivering it, let alone "dumping" it on unwilling ears.

Finally, your own emotional state and the pressure you are under at the time will influence how you practice. Being aware of your frame of mind and not rushing through the process can help keep your conversations collaborative and on target. Your heart needs to be in it—focused not on what you want, but on the well-being of the patient.

Avoid giving advice in the service of the righting reflex.

The Ask–Offer–Ask Framework

The Ask–Offer–Ask framework emerged originally from research on what makes for effective feedback of assessment results and was then adapted for wider use in health care. The three core activities (ask, offer, ask) are described below, and whether in sequence or in a more circular pattern, there is a to-and-fro rhythm involved that resembles closely the conversation patterns in MI itself.

Ask

If you are going to offer information or advice, it is often helpful to ask permission first, especially if the patient seems reluctant or uninterested. Then, if the patient agrees, engage with them and find out what they know or would like to know. Doing this not only helps set a collaborative tone for the conversation, but also saves time otherwise spent giving information the patient might already know. Examples of useful questions include: "How do you feel about . . . ?" "What do you already know or have tried?" "What would you really like to know about this?" Listening well here, even briefly, will be well worth it. Even at this stage, the patient often responds with self-motivating change talk, such as "Well, I already know that my smoking is terrible for my heart and lungs, but I guess what I really need is help in actually taking the plunge."

Offer

Present your idea as an informed suggestion, an offering rather than an instruction. Keep to facts if you can, and leave it to the patient to clarify their relevance. Stay positive and offer ideas about what to do rather than what not to do, for example, "Consider eating healthier food," rather than "Don't eat so much fatty food." Offer choice as much as possible. Use language like "might" rather than "should"; and "I wonder whether . . ." rather than "Something you really have to do is. . . . " You can see "offering" as akin to "showing," rather than "telling."

Ask

Here's the really productive moment: Ask the patient what they think about your advice or information, and listen for all you are worth, because here you might notice change talk and find yourself right in the heart of good MI practice. Useful questions include "What do you think of my suggestion?" "How does my idea fit with your plan?" "What will work the best or the worst here?" "How could you improve given what we've talked about?" "Could you see a way to fit any of this into your busy life right now?" "How does this information/advice fit into your everyday life?"

Ask–Offer–Ask in Everyday Practice

As you review the examples below, consider two key questions: Is it possible to be brief and efficient while spending a little more time on listening? Second, can giving advice and information be merged efficiently and effectively with MI?

EXAMPLE 1: Routine Feedback of a Test Result: Hospital Inpatient; Raising a Difficult Subject

Giving a routine test result all too often is viewed as the simple delivery of concrete information. But, for the person on the receiving end it might be anything but simple or concrete. How do you make the most out of a short exchange to ensure that the patient understands the feedback, absorbs the emotional impact, and can make good use of it? Seeing each patient as a unique person is a useful starting point. Ask–Offer–Ask can then be used to frame the conversation. Here's what it might look like:

> [*The patient has a gastric condition probably caused by excessive alcohol use. It is potentially a difficult personal issue for her to talk about.*]
>
> PRACTITIONER: (*Greets patient at bedside; introduces herself, engages briefly, and confirms that the person feels comfortable enough to chat.*) Yesterday they took blood from you, and although we haven't met before, is it okay if I give you the result of your liver test?
>
> PATIENT: Is it bad news?
>
> PRACTITIONER: Let's see what you think. It's a worry rather than a critical medical problem. The liver is a wonderful organ that can usually heal itself if you look after it right. Looking at your records, I see here that you sometimes use alcohol more than the recommended limits, you have this stomach problem, and I am curious to know how you see the link between drinking alcohol and your health? [*Ask*]
>
> PATIENT: Nothing really, other than that drinking too much is probably bad for the body. But, I don't often go over the top with drinking. [*Sustain talk*]
>
> PRACTITIONER: You're not sure about drinking and this test result. [*Listening statement*]
>
> PATIENT: Yes, that's right, what does it say?
>
> PRACTITIONER: See what you think about this. [*Switching to the Offer phase*] The result shows that the enzymes from your liver cells are raised in your blood. At these levels, this means that your liver is being damaged, but that it might not be too late to do something about it. Any thoughts? [*Shifting to the Ask phase*]
>
> PATIENT: Well, you are saying that my drinking is harming my liver? I don't drink any more than my friends. [*Sustain talk*]
>
> PRACTITIONER: You feel the results don't make sense. [*Listening statement*]
>
> PATIENT: Do I have to stay longer in the hospital now?
>
> PRACTITIONER: No, not because of your liver. I am thinking now of how you can make smart decisions going forward about your health, your stomach, and your liver.

PATIENT: Well, I'm shocked. [*Change talk*] Another doctor told me about drinking and my stomach, now you talk about the liver. The thing is we all drink like this. It's part of our social life and our work life, and at home my husband and I like to relax together each evening. [*Sustain talk*]

PRACTITIONER: And yet, you think the result may be a bit unfair on you given how much you drink. [*Listening statement*]

PATIENT: Yes, that's right. I don't drink all that much, but then I guess I don't want any more problems than I already have right now. This gut thing is bad enough. [*Change talk*]

PRACTITIONER: And, you are not sure about the link with alcohol. [*Listening statement*]

PATIENT: Not till now to be honest. I didn't realize that the amount I drink could be doing that to my liver. [*Change talk*]

PRACTITIONER: What if I give you some more time to rest now and think? I can drop by tomorrow morning, and we can chat a bit more then. I can also answer any questions you might have. (*Patient agrees.*)

How might that exchange have unfolded if the practitioner listened less and risked a more direct and confrontational approach to information delivery? What if the test result was something potentially more drastic for the patient, for example, an unexpected positive finding on an HIV test? A confrontational style usually elicits denial when it comes to difficult information or advice.

EXAMPLE 2: Routine Advice Giving—Primary Care

Advice is a step up in complexity from giving information because it contains a clear message about why or how the patient could change their behavior. Here's a common example, involving a patient who is a likable and talkative person: a heavy goods vehicle driver of around 55, overweight, and who smokes regularly.

PATIENT: So, you are saying my blood pressure is too high?

PRACTITIONER: It is quite high, yes, high enough for me to prescribe some medication right away.

PATIENT: I see.

PRACTITIONER: But before you leave, if I may, I just want to ask you about your lifestyle and offer you some advice here, too. [*Ask*]

PATIENT: Okay, what?

PRACTITIONER: Tell me first, how you feel about your health and what you know about high blood pressure? [*Ask*] (*Patient states what he knows about high blood pressure, and the practitioner continues.*) Yes, you have a pretty good understanding of what's going on. Can I offer you some advice?

PATIENT: Well sure, I'm not the sort of person to run away from life if you know what I mean. My son always says that I love giving advice to everyone else, but I hate being on the receiving end myself. But now I'm here, and I guess I must face the music.

PRACTITIONER: You want to keep healthy. [*Listening statement*]

PATIENT: Oh, for sure. I enjoy my life and I work hard also. I need to keep going for a few more years. (*Laughs.*) [*Change talk*]

PRACTITIONER: Let me make some suggestions now, and I want to make sure we talk about how you really feel about this because it's your choice how to proceed from here. I am here to back you up. You are the driver and I am sitting alongside you, if you know what I mean.

PATIENT: I think I get you. The trucks I drive are big, mind you. (*Laughs.*) What are you saying here?

PRACTITIONER: (*Offers advice about adjusting lifestyle, highlighting choices about what to tackle, whether it is diet, smoking, or exercise.*) So, these are your choices and, as I said, you are in the driver's seat. What do you think? What makes the most sense to you? [*Ask*]

PATIENT: Now that's a shock. [*Change talk*] What you are saying has big implications for me, all day, every day, given my job and all. The medicine won't do it by itself?

PRACTITIONER: It can help, but I wanted to be honest with you about also tackling your lifestyle.

PATIENT: Now you've got me. I usually have an answer to everything, but now I don't.

PRACTITIONER: You want to get your blood pressure under control. [*Listening statement*]

PATIENT: Well, of course, but this is pretty frightening to be honest. [*Change talk*]

PRACTITIONER: You are not sure what to do, yet you would like to get your blood pressure down. [*Listening statement*]

PATIENT: I guess I have no choice, really, when I think about it.

PRACTITIONER: (*Reminds him of choices and invites him to return.*) What do you say you talk it over with your family, and then come back in a week so we can discuss next steps, if this would seem helpful?

CONSIDER: A Practitioner Speaks

Before I learnt MI, advice giving was my default style in the main; that is what I was taught to do, and I thought it was my role. The Ask–Offer–Ask strategy developed in MI helped me find a way to do it skilfully because I give advice, almost every day, but I listen first and then again afterwards. What happens is that the patient starts telling me what they make of the advice, and before I know it, I can use MI to help them move forward. And, sometimes, I don't even have to do or say much because they say it all for themselves. It all just comes out. Not just the reasons why they plan to change, but concrete plans also often just flow, with me having suggested very little.

—JUDITH CARPENTER, *dietitian and MI trainer*

The examples above were straightforward, with the practitioners under minimal pressure. Then there are situations that, although less common, are more difficult to navigate because your information will be especially hard for the person to hear and adapt to, like telling someone they can no longer drive their car. Here, it can be useful to:

- Notice your own emotional state at the start and to prepare yourself mentally ahead of the difficult conversation.
- Pause to take a breath while you remind yourself of how you will approach the scenario.
- Consider slowing down the pace to give both you and the patient time to think.
- Proceed with an approach that is authentic, honest, and respectful of the person, yet also clear about the problem.
- Emphasize choice wherever possible.

Experienced clinicians often signal their intention by saying they have some important information to provide, and they gain the patient's agreement to do this by asking permission at the outset. The Ask–Offer–Ask framework can then be used to ensure that the patient is given the opportunity to digest the implications of your information.

Conclusion

We opened this chapter with questions about what skillful practice looks like and how this might be integrated with MI. A common conundrum presented by practitioners learning MI is what to do when patients from certain communities and cultures walk into the consulting room, "expecting to be told what to do," or "when I hear something that raises serious concern, I must intervene and advise, and I also want to be MI consistent." The Ask–Offer–Ask framework should enable you to address these dilemmas because you give both clear advice and empower the patient in the same conversation. It reminds us of this age-old saying:

> Tell me, and I will forget
> Show me, and I may remember
> Involve me, and I will understand.
> —XUN KUANG, *Confucian philosopher*

Seen in this light, the process is not merely a task but a skill set, requiring artistry to execute in a compassionate and effective manner.

CHAPTER 12

MI Briefly

Go alone go faster, go together go farther.
—An African Saying

I've got this long-term condition and I go in and out of the clinic,
see lots of different practitioners, wait around quite a lot, and
then some people stand out as special. That's what happened with
this nurse whom I met for just a minute or two when she checked
my weight and blood pressure. Then a week or so later there was
this serious panic moment, what felt like a big backward step
in my health. They always said to call if there was trouble, and
I remembered this nurse's first name and asked for her. What a
relief. She gave me this advice, but when I put the phone down I
realized that the advice was not new to me but she reassured me
and gave me so much hope on a call that lasted 2–3 minutes.
—Stephen Rollnick

Brief conversations about change occur naturally throughout health care,
planned or not, and conveying hope and kindness that sit at the heart of
good practice takes no time at all. Here are some common examples of
when short interactions can be beneficial:

- A routine consultation, and just before a patient leaves, you decide
  to address a lifestyle issue.
- This patient says he is not keen on a reducing his painkillers. Now
  what?
- He is in bed with lots of time, and you decide to have a brief chat
  about his control of blood sugars.
- Her weight is definitively an issue, let alone that of her child. This
  should be raised. But, how?

Can MI help you to improve these brief encounters and empower
people, even if you have just a minute or two? Our experience has been

that as you get more familiar with the skills involved in MI, you become more proficient at asking just the right question, making a helpful listening statement, or using a summary to pull things together sharply—and then moving on. The essence of doing MI well in brief conversations is a move away from a "find it, fix it" approach and messages like "This is what you need to do, let me tell you why and how." Rather, aim for an approach more like this: "I hear you, and would like to offer you some help. Here's where you might go. How do you see the road ahead?" Championing autonomy is a powerful vehicle for change and doesn't require any more time than the traditional directive approach.

> **Move away from a "find it, fix it" approach.**

Just a Minute or Two

What might a conversation informed by MI look like in a minute or two, even with someone who feels reluctant to change? *How* you do this will matter. A stern warning will usually not land as well as a message that inspires hope and confidence.

Consider this example below. It takes place in primary care, but the scenario could arise in other settings, too. The specifics of the presenting problem matter less than the challenge involved: raising a difficult subject and sowing the seeds for taking action to improve health and well-being.

EXAMPLE 1: Primary Care—A Difficult Subject

PRACTITIONER: Okay, this wound should heal if you keep it clean. Before you go, can I speak with you about something else that concerns me?

PATIENT: What's that?

PRACTITIONER: You say you got this wound in a fight last night down there in the village, yes?

PATIENT: Yes, I was lucky. He could have killed me.

PRACTITIONER: It could have been much worse for you. And with everyone drinking and shouting, you came out lucky. [*Listening statements*]

PATIENT: You just don't know what's going to happen down there sometimes.

PRACTITIONER: I guess that's also part of the fun. [*Listening statements*]

PATIENT: Not with the fighting. That was crazy.

PRACTITIONER: Can I ask you about something else, please? [*Asking permission*]

PATIENT: Sure, ask me anything.

PRACTITIONER: I have another concern about when you have been drinking. You might want to be careful of having sex without a condom because there is quite a lot of HIV out there at the moment, and that can be a bad infection to get.

PATIENT: No, it won't get me. I am careful.

PRACTITIONER: You have noticed some people getting sick and you don't want that. [*Listening statement*]

PATIENT: Yes, I don't want that. [*Change talk*]

PRACTITIONER: This is your choice. You can always come back to me for an HIV test if you want to, okay? I would advise you to do this so you know because if you are infected, there is medicine that can keep you healthy.

PATIENT: Thank you. I will think about this. [*Change talk*]

What MI offers is an avenue for sowing the seed that is as free as possible from discord and discomfort, while nevertheless enabling the practitioner to get a message across that makes best use of precious time during busy routine practice. Besides a willingness to be authentic and compassionate and to offer hope, the practitioner in the above exchange made listening statements that, in turn, evoked some change talk. This won't happen every time. Some people might be feeling more defensive than the patient in the example above. However, using a foundation of compassionate communication will ensure that planting a seed can be achieved without undue conflict.

Ten Minutes or More

What about somewhat longer chats? Taking 10–15 minutes or more to offer brief advice about the benefits of change is often called "brief intervention." It's sometimes preceded by screening, and is most commonly focused on topics like smoking, alcohol use, and other lifestyle behaviors. Here, the African saying that opened this chapter is well worth adhering to: "Go alone go faster, go together go

MI offers an avenue for sowing the seed for taking action, without creating discord.

farther." When using MI as a brief intervention, your mindset is focused on change, like going on a walk, where you invite the patient to go down the path of change, curious about why and how they think they might achieve this, and ready to offer information and advice as needed.

A Framework for Brief MI

Figure 12.1 presents a framework for how you might use MI briefly. You will notice the four processes, and how information and advice giving can be seamlessly integrated into the conversation (see Chapter 11). The core skills of MI are used throughout the journey. We placed the summary at the end, aware also that you can use a summary at any point, perhaps to clarify things or to regain some control of the direction of the consultation.

EXAMPLE 2: Hospital Outpatient—Lifestyle Review

Here is a narrative account of a fictional consultation in a routine outpatient clinic, where the map in Figure 12.1 served as a guideline. A moment arose when it became clear that talking about lifestyle change might be valuable. This cheerful man of 52 was holding down a job as a casual laborer, supporting a large family, living in relative poverty in dense inner-city housing. His case notes revealed concern about poor

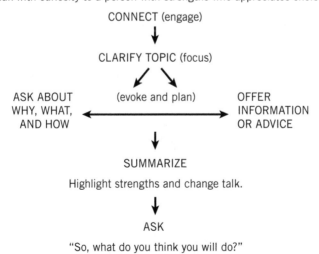

FIGURE 12.1. Brief MI framework.

glycemic control, his belief that medication could solve his diabetes problem for him, and the potential threat of smoking and poor diet to his health.

"I felt that our rapport was good enough to risk asking him about his lifestyle, even though he seemed to imagine that medicine was all he really needed from the hospital. The discussion took a total of 15 minutes, and I started by following that '20% rule' [see Chapter 7]: just listen for roughly the first 20% of the consultation time [ENGAGE]. I asked permission to talk about his lifestyle and diabetes [FOCUS], and chose a single open question to start us off: 'How do you see the links between your diabetes and your lifestyle, the way you eat, the exercise you get and that sort of thing?' I steered away from asking investigative questions like 'How much do you smoke?' He mentioned right away that he had been told about his smoking and diet, and I simply used listening statements in reply, with a clear focus on his experience and strengths. He seemed proud of how fit he was as a laborer.

"Then I switched direction [FOCUS] and asked him, 'How do you see the best way to keep healthy in the years to come?' Again, this was where listening statements helped [EVOKE]. It turned out that he was concerned to some degree about his smoking but didn't feel able or confident to quit or to do anything really but keep going and cope with life as it unfolded. I just tried to understand how he felt about change.

"When I summarized what he told me, he seemed appreciative. I decided to ask about the what and the how more specifically: 'If you were to take just a few steps forward, what do you think you might do?' [PLAN] He seemed at a loss, so I offered him some options using the Ask–Offer–Ask framework [see Chapter 11]. He agreed to think about them and we arranged a follow-up appointment 2 weeks later."

Using MI briefly is greatly aided by the use of one or two evocative questions that hand the baton over to the patient to say why and how they might change (see Chapter 9 on evoking).

Managing Time and the Value of Listening

It's an experience that many practitioners report to us: The more skilled you get with MI, the less time it takes. Put another way, as you develop restraint and avoid stepping in with distracting questions and unsolicited advice, choices open up for you to make the most of the time available. Open questions give you time to think and to feel less rushed. Practitioners who succeed in consulting without feeling rushed talk about "being in a zone" where time all but stands still. Patients also report a similar experience, of feeling satis-fied in a brief consultation where the practi-tioner seemed to be in no rush at all. A good consultation feels like you took longer than you actually did.

MI allows you and the patient to get the most of a brief consultation.

CONSIDER: Listening Saves Time—A Clinician Speaks

He's been someone I have been working with for years. He was at a major crossroad in his life, with advanced renal disease, and he had absolutely refused to consider dialysis even though I had this relationship with him. I've been very worried about him. I didn't want to lose him to a medical illness. I realized I hadn't been really engaging him afresh every time I met him. What came to mind was the reminder to really listen to him about what he was feeling; and the need to reflect, just reflect, really reflect. So, I went back and started engagement anew, and this time it was within about 5–10 minutes, he opened up his heart, and within a few minutes he had this change talk. He said, "I want to go back and see the renal physician," and it was really a breakthrough. Within about 10–15 minutes he was out of my room. Our normal consultations would be 20 minutes to half an hour. He felt good, I felt good. The use of listening with reflections saved me time. He was able to bring in the focus himself. We were both very calm and it was quick and fast.

—NG MIN YIN, MD

Conclusion

To use MI briefly requires a keen sense of the patient's potential, and a clear mind. Much of the skill comes from an awareness of what not to say, what to leave out. With that mindset, it is possible to do a lot in a short time.

CHAPTER 13

MI and Assessment

The quality of assessors is critical to the quality
of the assessment result.

—PEARL ZHU

Imagine your clinic's management signals a new era with another assessment system with a set of questions to ask every patient at the start of the consultation, and to be checked off on the desktop computer. You want to bring MI into your everyday practice, knowing engagement at the start of a consultation is fundamental to good practice. Now what? The battery of questions might suit the new system, but it looks as if it will depress engagement. Increasing numbers of practitioners are faced with variations of this challenge, where the system seems of higher priority than developing trust and connection.

Not every clinic will operate like this one, but the issue comes up, whatever assessment procedure is used: How do you conduct assessment while retaining the interest and engagement of the patient, let alone bring MI skills and the mindset of a guide into the consultation? How do you establish a conversation between equals, rather than proceeding as an authority figure conducting a one-way question-asking session?

A Dynamic Exchange

Can assessment involve a two-way exchange? From the early 1980s, efforts were made to integrate MI with assessment, when Miller and colleagues hit on a simple realization that has borne the test of time: Instead of telling patients what assessment data and test results about them meant, practitioners asked them to indicate how they saw the data and test results. Outcomes were better all round, and this gave rise to the Ask–Offer–Ask framework (described in Chapter 11), stimulating colleagues to explore ways of moving, as one of them put it, "from checklists to conversations."[*] Just one or two simple open questions can tilt a potentially disengaging assessment into an empowering conversation. The examples below all illustrate this ability to get the best out of assessment without losing the engagement and evoking that give MI its impetus. No question, integrating MI with assessment involves a mind-set change for the practitioner, a move away from the mechanistic view of gathering information to one of really listening and connecting while you conduct an assessment.

Formal Assessment

If you need to conduct a formal assessment, consider enhancing engagement by spending a minute or two in conversation first. Listen to what a patient is wanting from the consultation, and then ask permission to shift direction to assessment. Patients usually go along with this quite readily. For example, "It sounds like what matters the most to you is to get some help with (a problem). Before we do just this, from my side I need to complete this assessment, and I wonder if it's okay for me to take you through **Before assessment, spend** this now?" You can also prompt patients to **a minute or two enhancing** look out for topics or questions to ask you **engagement.** about afterward.

Having completed the assessment, you can enter the evoking process quite rapidly with curious open questions, leading to the kind of dynamic exchange that takes you right into MI territory. Useful questions include:

"What did you notice that you were curious about?"

"If I point to that blood result which was abnormal, what do you make of this?"

"Most people have a systolic blood pressure around 100 or at most 120, whereas yours was well over 140. I wonder how you feel about this."

---

[*]We thank Kylie McKenzie, who suggested this useful phrase to us.

Informal Assessment and Diagnosis

Short-answer and closed questions serve a useful function when fact finding, but do they have the unintended consequence of undermining engagement, and at what cost? For decades, the teaching of assessment and diagnosis in health care education involved training students to ask one closed question after another, leaving many to continue this tradition throughout their careers. While some clinical problems require this focused approach, most do not. A more integrated and patient-centered approach to assessment has been emerging, championed by clinicians who interweave closed questions with open ones in a two-way exchange. Information is gathered with closed questions, and open questions are used to encourage the patient to elaborate. For example:

PRACTITIONER: Hello. Can I call you, Mr. Lloyd?

PATIENT: No, Jim is fine, thank you.

PRACTITIONER: You look in some pain, Jim. [*Listening statement*]

PATIENT: It's my back over here.

PRACTITIONER: I will examine you in a moment, but tell me: What happened? [*Open question*]

PATIENT: Last week I was just bending down to put the lead on the dog, and bang . . . my back went and I couldn't straighten up. The pain was excruciating. I have never had this before.

PRACTITIONER: You were heading out for exercise. [*Listening statement*]

PATIENT: Yes, I hate it, but it has to happen with a dog.

PRACTITIONER: Show me again exactly where this pain is. (*Asks three more closed questions about location.*) What has helped to relieve the pain since last week? [*Open question*]

PATIENT: Lying down is very good, and I can sit in the chair with a cushion behind me, but when I move suddenly, that's the problem.

PRACTITIONER: So, you've been experimenting and have noticed what helps. [*Affirmation*]

PATIENT: Yes, I can walk okay as long as it's slowly.

PRACTITIONER: So, I wonder what questions you might have for me now. [*Open question*]

PATIENT: Are you saying that my back will get better?

The interweaving of questions with other core skills brings about a comfortable rhythm to the consultation that is both efficient from an assessment point of view and engaging for both participants. The use of open questions also allows you a little breathing space to observe and bring the best of MI to the fore because you have time to notice things the patient says that provide the openings for raising the subject of lifestyle change. In the prior example, the practitioner noticed the patient's comment about walking the dog, and the following short exchange (involving a guiding style and MI) could have emerged directly from the assessment:

Using open questions allows you breathing space to observe.

PRACTITIONER: You mentioned walking the dog. . . . Speaking of exercise, building up muscle strength in your lower back could be important for protecting you from pain going forward. I wonder how you might develop some exercise habits that you enjoy and look forward to.

PATIENT: Walking the dog is not one them. In fact, she is so big that she drags me along and this just makes me feel stressed, to be honest. [*Sustain talk*]

PRACTITIONER: It's not relaxing for you. [*Listening statement*]

PATIENT: I'm also not the type to go to the gym even if I could afford it. [*Sustain talk*]

PRACTITIONER: That won't work for you. [*Listening statement*]

PATIENT: Are you saying I must do this to sort out this pain?

PRACTITIONER: It's your choice here. Exercise is one really helpful way of preventing further problems with your back. Maybe you would prefer to exercise with someone, I don't know.

PATIENT: Okay, I'll talk to my son because he often finds a way to get me off my sofa. [*Change talk*]

PRACTITIONER: You can see that working for you, one small step that could help to get you going. [*Listening statement*]

PATIENT: Yes, I will definitely have a word with him. [*Change talk*]

Hearing the Patient's Story: A Typical Day

A quite different approach to assessment and diagnosis can be found in the use of a strategy we first developed with a hospital for patients with high levels of alcohol consumption (Rollnick, Heather, & Bell, 1992). It requires 5–7 minutes, is entirely patient-driven, and is particularly useful early on in a consultation.

This strategy, which we call "A Typical Day," is built on something we noticed skilled practitioners doing routinely: asking the patient to tell their story. It can be adapted to any setting—in our case, we wanted to know where alcohol fit into their lives, how much they drank, and how this might be affecting them, all of which are questions usually asked in a formal assessment. But instead of starting the consultation with this assessment of alcohol use, which risked eliciting a defensive reaction, we asked patients to *take around 5–7 minutes to walk us through a typical day in their lives*. We took great care *not* to ask investigative questions. Even if the patient mentioned little about alcohol, we found that the investment of our time and genuine interest in their lives allowed us to raise the subject of alcohol use in an easy manner immediately afterward. Indeed, we were able to fill in the blanks of our assessment with a few closed questions without difficulty. Here are the key guidelines:

1. Invite the person to take you through a typical day in their life. If needed, help them to locate one. Clarify the purpose, which is to understand what everyday life is like for them. *Adopt a curious mindset and remind yourself not to interfere by zoning in on any issue or problem.*
2. Start at the beginning of the day and focus on the patient's behavior and how they felt. They woke up. Then what did they do, and how did they feel?
3. As their story unfolds, you might ask them to give you some more detail here and there, or to speed up or slow down.
4. Once they have finished, ask the patient if they would like to add anything to their story.

This strategy not only enhances engagement but also aids assessment because as the patient's story unfolds, all sorts of details emerge about their behavior, mood, the pressures on them, and where openings for improving their health might lie. It is like imagining they are painting a picture on a blank canvas, and this is their opportunity to fill the canvas with the colors of their choice. Over the following decades, we were able to adapt this strategy for use in other areas, and in other forms, like asking a patient to take you through a typical episode of pain from start to finish, or telling you how a typical evening meal evolves.

Using the "A Typical Day" strategy not only enhances engagement but also aids assessment.

Conclusion

Asking patients for some information is a normal part of health care. A common approach is to ask for "just the facts" by going through a decision tree of closed questions, at the end of which you prescribe an answer. However, when what is needed is a change in the person's behavior or lifestyle, this Question–Answer–Prescription approach is seldom effective. You need your patient's active engagement in the conversation to find their own motivation for and ideas about healthy change. Yes, it may take a few minutes longer, but the effect can be enduring. Similarly, when you want to offer information or advice, it is usually more effective to do so in a collaborative way that includes asking for and listening to your patient's own perspectives.

CHAPTER 14

MI in Groups

Don't do for a group what a group can do for itself.
—EMILY M. AXELROD

Dixie was one of the quiet ones in the group, and you would have bet on her *not* making a decision to change. All she had said was that she lacked confidence to meet with friends and get more exercise. Then the next week she turned up having made progress. "You kind people helped me to think this through in the group, and I got the courage to have a go. I went for a walk with my best friend."

That's a common story of someone who felt inspired by others in a supportive group. She had felt the empathy of others and the freedom to make up her own mind about what to do. Her motivation was lifted by simply hearing others talk and reflecting about what she might do. Such is the healing power of a group that is working well.

Using MI in a group takes the idea of a support group one step further with a specific focus on encouraging its participants' change talk, their own good reasons to change. The facilitator holds back from persuading patients to change and purposefully steers the conversation away from talk about problems to giving even the quieter people the chance to say out loud why and how they might make positive changes. Just as it does in a consultation with a single patient, this change talk in a group can be a powerful expression of motivation for and action toward change.

MI can be used in an educational group or a support group, either in person or online. This chapter provides a broad overview as well as details about setting up a group, running it, and some of the nuances involved along the way. It assumes a basic understanding of MI, as outlined in Chapter 2, and familiarity with the skills involved (see Part II). You can find well-worked examples of MI in health care groups in Lane, Butterworth, and Speck (2013) and Steinberg and Miller (2015).

The most common concern we hear from both patients and practitioners in a group is a feeling of being potentially overwhelmed by the experience because you never really know what someone might come up with and whether things could get a bit out of control. A commonly used solution is to structure the meeting tightly to ensure safety, and simply to provide educational material for all to discuss. MI provides a middle ground between tight structure and open discussion, rooted in the style of a guide. You remain in charge of the structure and process; you might offer expert information and advice, but your main focus is helping participants to say what change might mean for them. It's a positive, forward-looking discussion, fed by the use of core skills that maximize their active involvement. Remember that evoking and listening to patients' own change talk are key. You can explore this topic in greater detail in Wagner and Ingersoll (2013) and find useful strategies with examples in Lane and colleagues (2013). We start with how a patient education group can be made consistent with MI, and then turn to the wider use of MI whether or not there is an educational component.

> **MI in a group focuses on encouraging participant change talk.**

> **MI allows a middle ground for group work, between a tight structure and open discussion.**

Patient Education Groups

It is possible to run patient education group meetings that are MI-consistent. Indeed, what the use of MI highlights is that it is not just the transmission of information that makes for good outcomes, but how patients make sense of it. This opens up considerable room for innovation. Our suggestion is to use the Ask–Offer–Ask framework described in Chapter 11 in which translation into a group setting is straightforward.

CONSIDER: An Online Educational Group

We gathered a group of patients online for an educational session about getting a COVID vaccine. There were 31 patients on the call, and we used the Ask–Offer–Ask strategy which gave people time to ask questions. The discussion then flowed smoothly around topics like side effects, infertility and genetic mutation. A questionnaire administered afterwards revealed satisfaction with the session and around 20% of the participants felt more confident about taking the vaccine.

—ALESSANDRO DIANA, MD

The box that follows offers an overview of how this Ask–Offer–Ask framework would look in a patient education setting.

Ask–Offer–Ask: Tips for Groups

Using the Ask–Offer–Ask framework provides a structure that allows you to engage patients and highlight areas for improvement both before and after a period of offering information (see Chapter 11 for details). Outcomes are likely to improve when you use this framework.

TOP TIPS

1. Inform patients about ground rules (see details below).
2. Avoid urging participants to change—that's for them to decide.
3. After presenting information, ask them what the implications are.

INTRODUCTION

Welcome people, particularly new members. Clarify ground rules, for example: No one needs to speak; the aim is to learn about the topic, and to help each other make positive changes. State the topic for the meeting, ideally in the form of a question, such as "How can exercise help us?" No need for audio or visual aids to begin with.

ASK

Give this phase of the session quality time, up to one-third of the meeting. Select one or more open questions to ask the group about the topic, for example, "Who would like to begin?" "What would you most like to know about [the topic]?" "What concerns do you have about [the topic]?" "What questions do you have about [the topic]?" Your main challenge at this point is to keep the focus on the chosen topic and question. You can make the transition to the next phase by summarizing what's been offered up by group members.

OFFER

Make just a few key points, up to about three. If you use a visual aid, try to tell a story about a patient to illustrate these points. Clarify the facts, and try to not use threatening, dogmatic, or fear-filled language, such as "So, if you don't be careful, you could end up having a stroke." Rather, say something like "This can put people at a much higher risk for stroke." Switch off visual aids.

ASK

Signal that it is group members' time to talk. Useful questions include: "What did you make of that information?" "What struck you as most relevant to you?" "What questions do you have about this topic?" "What one or two points did you pick up from the presentation?" "What improvements might you make in your everyday life?" "What would a healthier you look and feel like?"

Setting Up a Group

We turn now to the conduct of a group that has a wider scope or purpose than a purely educational group: to help patients learn from each other and improve their health. Your goal will be to merge patient empowerment and education into a satisfying experience for all. A good place to start is often by speaking with colleagues and patient themselves. Get their input in formulating the group objectives using such questions as:

- *What is the aim of the group?* This is essential to clarify first.
- *Will this be an open or closed group?* There are pros and cons on your side and theirs.
- *Will the group be designed with a fixed length, or will it be ongoing? What will participants and you find most convenient?*
- *What time of day is best to hold the group meetings?*
- *Would participants enjoy informal time with tea or coffee before or afterward?*
- *Who will facilitate the meetings? Which colleagues have experience in group facilitation?* Often it is best to work in pairs.
- *How many participants should we invite initially?* Some initial nonattendance is likely.

With these decisions in place, even tentatively, and a willingness to monitor, adjust, and take feedback from patients, what might a group based on MI look and feel like?

Running a Group

To run an MI-consistent group well, it is advisable to have someone on the team with a degree of competence in group facilitation. Working as a pair of facilitators is good practice, taking care to clarify who will lead the group, and what helpful and less helpful support to each other will look like.

What follows below are the principles and practice that emerged from groups we ran that worked well in a hospital outpatient setting. Some of the features, like establishing and expressing ground rules, will be common to all successful MI-informed groups. Other features might need tweaking to suit your circumstances. Our experience comes from working with patients with a long-term condition, like diabetes, and heart, kidney, or respiratory diseases.

Opening a Meeting

We found the four processes highlighted in this book to be useful when running groups. As it is when treating individuals, engagement is a top priority when beginning groups, and we have used a range of strategies for arranging seating, welcoming group members, and helping with introductions.

An opening statement and reminder of the aim of the meeting are well worth starting with routinely. Keep this simple, saying, for example, "As a reminder, our goals for these meetings are to support each other to make positive change in everyday life; to find out more about your conditions; and to enjoy chatting together."

At the start of each meeting, we also restate ground rules for the group (you may want to set some of your own):

1. Give everyone a chance to speak.
2. You are not obliged to speak.
3. We talk about challenges with a focus on positive solutions.

These ground rules are not only useful to help patients feel safe but they also provide security for facilitators: If you notice a guideline being violated at some point in the meeting, you can intervene and remind the group of the guideline in a positive manner. For example, a patient does little but describe problems and how difficult things are for them, leaving others feeling down or anxious. You can then gently remind the person of the meeting's aims and guidelines and steer the discussion in a positive direction.

Engagement is a top priority in beginning a group.

Getting Going

Most group leaders will kick off a meeting with a simple warm-up open question, like "How are you doing today?" This opening question is designed to help people relax, start chatting, and say what they think and feel (engaging). If you imagine the conversation as a balloon being tossed around among participants, your open question is an invitation to them to tap it around gently among themselves, rather than bash it back fearfully, or send it straight back your way. Group members do most of the talking.

Talking About Change

Whether a patient education session or a more open-ended group meeting, you can create the opportunity to encourage talk about change (focusing and evoking), and this is where MI skills come to the fore. The most widely used strategy is to ask open questions, the answer to which is change talk (evoking). For example, "Turning to the future, what have you noticed that could be of help to you going forward?", "How might you begin to enjoy exercise more?", or "What else has been particularly useful for you personally?" This is when you will hear the kind of change talk highly likely to predict better outcomes. In the supportive atmosphere you have created, even that quiet member might be bold enough to speak up at this point. The rhythm of exchange involves a facilitator asking a question, holding back from giving advice or having lengthy one-to-one conversations with individuals, and encouraging others to come up with their own ideas about what might work well for them and others.

Common Challenges

A unique challenge in groups arises when one member gives advice to another in a strong and pointed manner that makes the receiver feel defensive or cornered; for example, "Why don't you just make a decision and stick to it? I found it helpful to get my wife to remind me every day." This occurs most often when talking about action (planning). For someone who is feeling ambivalent, just as in individual consultations, this kind of intervention is not necessarily helpful. As facilitator, you can try a number of approaches to address this issue: Offer a reflection or open question to gently redirect the focus, for example, "You are trying to be helpful here, and I wonder what else might be useful?" Ask other group members for suggestions; you might emphasize how what works for some might not work for others; or you can use the linking summary mentioned below.

Another very common challenge is when patients talk about how difficult it is to change; in other words, what you hear is not change talk but sustain talk. This is perfectly normal and need not be a problem as long as it does not overwhelm the group or an individual in it. In one group, we developed a ground rule, "Keep problem talk to a minimum," to highlight the value of talking positively about change. Sometimes, however, patients say things when they feel downhearted or frustrated that stand out as not leading anywhere constructive, unless you intervene in some way.

Consider how you might respond to a group member who expresses sustain talk like this: "All I ever do is put on more weight, and I am getting tired of the nurses telling me to lose weight." In situations like this, we would see an opportunity to shift the discussion around in a positive direction. You surely would not want to hear time spent complaining about "those nurses" or a discussion that goes around in circles, with everyone simply saying how hard it is to change (i.e., loading up on sustain talk). So, how might you respond to encourage a more forward-facing and positive discussion? Consider the optional responses below, all guided by a belief in the strengths and wisdom of the group to really support each other. We list responses that might succeed in turning the discussion around in a positive direction, facing forward, toward change and responses that probably won't.

Ask a question, holding back from giving advice, and let others come up with their own ideas about what might work.

Recall, the patient says, "All I ever do is put on more weight, and I am getting tired of the nurses telling me to lose weight."

Helpful response choices

- "You don't like to be nagged, and you would like to find a way forward."
- "Despite this frustration, you came here today to see how you might make progress."
- "How would you like the nurses to help you?"
- "I bet there are other members of the group who would also like to find a way to lose weight and keep it down."
- "Can anyone tell us a story about succeeding with weight loss?"

Less helpful response choices

- "The nurses are only really wanting the best for you."
- "I bet there are other members of the group who also feel frustrated about trying to lose weight."

The helpful responses listed above have one thing in common: They call for change talk, and this ability to use a guiding style to steer the group conversation toward the positive is a hallmark of MI in a group. Some of those helpful responses are directed at individual patients, others at the group as a whole. The latter is important because what you are looking for is group members talking in a helpful way to each other, offering their reflections and stories. (Effectively, this would be evoking in a group.) That balloon metaphor mentioned earlier is worth bearing in mind. Your use of core skills enables participants to tap the balloon around between themselves.

Linking Summaries

A strategy unique to groups is the use of a summary that links people's contributions in a helpful way. Exchanges between group members can sometimes range far and wide, with even the occasional unhelpful remark here and there. What might be called a "linking summary" allows you to regain control, even to add a useful open question at the end of the summary to shift the focus in a more positive direction, for example, "There have been quite a lot of ideas offered here. Some of you feel a bit down about your progress, while others are trying to be helpful. Can I ask you all, what's the most helpful positive thing you are noticing here this evening?" You won't want to ignore or suppress problem talk (i.e., sustain talk), but that kind of linking summary helps you to find a better balance. If the discussion is heading in an unhelpful direction, you can always remind group members of the key guidelines: "We talk about challenges with a focus on positive solutions."

Useful Strategies and Adjustments

One strategy that can work well is to use a "round-robin" exercise when addressing a specific question. You ask participants to go around in circle, one at a time, and offer up their answer, giving them permission to "pass" if they so wish. Steinberg and Miller (2015) also describe other useful adjustments well worth exploring, for example, individual thinking time, and dividing up participants into dyads and triads.

MI in a group does not have to rely just on verbal exchanges. One striking practical exercise involves using the importance and confidence strategy (see Chapter 9), in which members are asked to place a rating of themselves on a whiteboard, thus allowing patients to notice how motivation to change varies, and giving the facilitator an opportunity to elicit change talk from participants with further open questions. This and other examples of useful activities and exercises can be found in Martino and Santa Ana (2013).

Closing the Meeting

If first impressions matter, so do last ones. Winding up a group meeting is a chance for participants to feel supported and connected to each other. There is also a chance to use MI to highlight and summarize those

If first impressions matter, so do last ones.

elements of the discussion that reflected the aim of the group, the useful ideas and decisions that emerged. For example:

> "Our time is now up, and the two of us want to thank you for coming here this evening, and especially to [name] for giving me my best laugh of the day! More seriously though, there was some heartfelt discussion about everyday challenges, and some particularly useful ideas about what it means to get on top of things like how small changes in daily routines can make such a big difference to the way you feel and to your health, too. It felt inspiring to hear how no one is really alone when it comes to having this condition. We will be around now for a few minutes if you want to have a word, so good night and all power to your friendship with and support to each other. See you same time next week."

Giving time to facilitators to debrief afterward is usually a marker of good practice.

Conclusion

Using patient groups offers a route to helping participants feel safe with each other, willing to say what they think and feel, supported by others and not sidelined into defensiveness by criticism, judgment, and a lack of acceptance. Not only are group visits more time-efficient, they add an important component of comradery and mutual support. Once participants do feel safe, the potential for learning new things and for making remarkable change is not an uncommon experience. What MI in a group adds is an ability to listen, steer, and affirm in such a way that participants voice their motivations and plans for change. Better outcomes will be there for all to witness.

CHAPTER 15

MI Remotely

Empathy is simply listening, holding space, withholding judgment,
emotionally connecting, and communicating that incredibly
healing message of you're not alone.

—Brene Brown

A few years back, we asked participants in a training workshop to let us know if they had interesting experiences on their return to everyday practice. One practitioner sent us this report: "I saw a client this morning via video who is profoundly deaf and a sign language user, and I spotted the change talk, reflected this back to her and the translator, and the change talk continued. A great moment."

In 2020, the COVID-19 pandemic caught the world by surprise, dramatically transforming social interaction. Essential services ordinarily provided in person were delivered remotely whenever possible. Health care practitioners, teachers, clergy, and businesses suddenly had to find new ways to provide services. Necessity led to discovery as telehealth became normal. But of course, this practice had been emerging for years before the pandemic hit, and anyone involved on the frontline will know of experiences like this:

- "It's different over the phone, more interrupting to begin with and then you learn how to handle pauses."
- "I'm not used to seeing my own face when I talk to someone."
- "When his face appeared on screen, it was fuzzy and there was a lag in the sound, too. And, we were there to talk about a difficult situation he was facing."

- "These young people are great at quick texts and emojis, but saying how they feel via text is trickier."
- "I was on time, so was he, and there he was in the supermarket, apparently looking forward to the call."

Such can be the pitfalls of remote consulting. While reading this book, one might ask, "Can MI be used remotely, too?" The simple answer is "yes," as long as you don't discard the relationship-driven quality that defines it. Indeed, if you don't want patients to be left behind by technology, the use of MI can protect both you and them from a mechanized and depersonalized approach to clinical practice. Comparison between MI delivered in person or via telephone yields similar outcomes (Boccio et al., 2017), and we counted over 20 studies that addressed the efficacy of MI over the telephone. These studies do not present an argument for discarding face-to-face consulting. Clinical experience will soon demand greater flexibility. Consider this recent example from a clinic we observed:

PRACTITIONER: (*Telephoning to inquire about adherence to thyroid medication*) Hello . . . Mrs. Jones? This is Dr. Walters. I'm calling from the clinic to chat with you about that blood test you came down for last week. (*Silence*) Mrs. Jones? Are you there? (*Silence*) Oh, we must have been cut off. (*Switches off phone.*)

PRACTITIONER: [*Second call*] Hello, Mrs. Jones, we might have been cut off. It's Dr. Walters again, forgive me for disturbing you. How are you? (*Silence again*) Mrs. Jones, are you there? (*Silence again, switches off phone.*)

PRACTITIONER: [*Third call*] Hello. Mrs. Jones, are you there?

PATIENT: (*Very quietly*) Yes.

PRACTITIONER: Oh, that's a relief, I thought we had been cut off. You might be feeling unwell, I am not sure. [*Listening statement*]

PATIENT: (*Silence, then*) Yes.

PRACTITIONER: Thank you for taking the call. I can tell this is not easy for you. [*Listening statement*]

PATIENT: It's not easy. I'm tired.

PRACTITIONER: And, you are not feeling like your usual self. [*Listening statement*]

The value of listening in that exchange is hard to miss. And telephone consulting? It was clearly of limited value on this occasion, and a face-to face conversation was the obvious next step, for assessing her condition and for that tricky conversation about medication adherence. A blended approach, in which remote and face-to-face consulting are used interchangeably, would seem well advised.

Who Wants What?

What guides the best decisions about using media like texts, telephone, and video consultations? Reaching large numbers is just one criterion. Efficiency is another. Practitioner well-being seems to feature also, as reflected in this coffee room remark by a nurse who said, "I like this telephone consulting. It's not only efficient, but I don't have the pressure of people waiting impatiently in the waiting room. Makes the day much easier to manage."

And, the patients? They are the most important factor to consider. If a person is about to speak about personal matters, what will suit them best? Young people like texting. Older people are new to it. While some prefer the telephone to a clinic visit, others feel exactly the opposite— the trip out to see a caring practitioner is uplifting and comforting. Not everyone has a computer and video, and the more marginalized the community, the less access they will have. Then there is clinical care and better outcomes. Since the aim of health care is to serve people's needs, any decision to rely on a single medium is bound to fall short of good practice.

Remote Consulting and MI: Skillful Practice

Remote consulting varies on a spectrum that runs from a patient's reading on the Internet and interacting with a robot at the one end, through texting, telephone consulting, and video consulting, before you get to the traditional face-to-face consultation at the other end of the spectrum. Where does MI fit in? It comes down to this: If a conversation prompts someone to consider why and how they might change, it starts to resemble consistency with MI. How might the use of MI improve the conduct of remote conversations?

> Relying on a single communication medium is bound to fall short of good practice.

Premature Action Talk and the Righting Reflex

The use of MI trains a practitioner to be mindful of jumping in too fast, especially with premature talk about changing this or that behavior when patients feel neither engaged nor given space to make up their own minds. Remote consulting is vulnerable here, like when a practitioner is obliged to call a list of patients with a long-term condition to discuss their progress. In the name of efficiency, it can be tempting just to make sure you ask the required series of questions about a patient's progress and lifestyle. This "questionnaire" approach is clearly some distance from what good practice looks like (see Chapter 12 for guidelines and tips about the brief consultation). The spirit of MI (see Chapter 2) calls attention to the foundations of good practice. Lose this spirit and patients will suffer.

A Finely Tuned Engaging Process

Texting, telephone, or video consulting highlights the need for even more skillful engaging. That's because in such conversations you can find patients in a wide range of contexts and environments—meaning there is no shortage of distractions, disruptions, and even ruptures to the engaging process. Practitioners routinely pick up a lot of information as patients walk into their consulting rooms—the way they walk, look, what they are carrying, and even their smell. This goes both ways: Patients will search for cues about your trustworthiness.

Engaging requires special attention when you are working remotely.

However, with remote consulting, you face the loss of such cues. Engaging is therefore a finely tuned process requiring special attention in its own right.

CONSIDER: Texting in Difficult Times

Over the last 3 months I have been in conversation with 100+ people who text for help through a crisis line, mostly in their teens or early twenties, and all in the middle of the night. I am not as fast as them in responding to messages, but while a small percentage drop away, it has mostly been possible to connect and engage, in hugely challenging circumstances. Many are feeling the impact of anxiety and panic attacks, others are simply feeling desperate, some are suicidal. It's a challenge to read the emotional tone of what sits behind just a few words. Yet people want to try and say how they feel if you give them a chance to engage. Put another way, if they don't feel they can trust you, they will not continue an open dialogue and your good intentions will amount to very little.

—Tony Rao, MD

Following are some pointers to good practice that we have encountered.

Clarify the Purpose

Explain at the outset why you are calling, what you plan to talk about, and how much time you have. This sets some expectations and prepares the patient for the conversation ahead. *Note:* If you are new to remote consulting, you can be put off your stride by intrusions and distractions. Get used to seeing your face up on a screen, make sure you have a quiet private place to hold remote appointments, and keep down background noise.

Make Use of Pauses

It's common to stumble a bit with awkward pauses when there is cross-talk and uncertainty about whose turn it is to talk next, like your brain is trying to "catch up" with what's going on. You can make good use of pauses as opportunities to double-check with the patient that you are on the same page—for example, "It is different talking like this on the telephone. How are you finding it? Have I understood you well enough? Is there anything I have missed?" Or, "You grew silent just now. What are you feeling?" If you have to pause to make notes or check your records, say so.

Be More Verbally Responsive Than You Would Be in an In-Person Consultation

Realize that your patient is also listening carefully to you without the usual benefit of in-person clues, especially on the telephone. Acknowledge at the outset that you intend to listen carefully. Provide reflections or short summaries a bit more often than you might in person. Offer more verbal affirmations. Remember that if you're on a telephone call, **Verbally convey your authentic presence and caring.** patients can't see you smiling or nodding your head, so communicate these gestures with your voice instead. Convey your authentic presence and caring through your words and vocalizations.

Evoking with Skill

With empathic listening at the heart of MI, your curious open questions and listening statements can be harnessed to good effect. Indeed, there is evidence that voice-only interaction can *increase* empathic accuracy (Kraus, 2017). You can focus more intently on the conversation. Ample information about meaning and experience are contained not only in the words themselves, but in the rich cues that accompany language: the volume, pitch, modulation, cadence, pauses, and fluency of speech. These cues do not require special training to detect because they are normally learned through social development interacting with others. For some patients consulting via telephone or video can even facilitate a degree of anonymity and honesty relative to face-to-face contact. For some practitioners consulting in this way can enhance their MI skill, evident in the story about a deaf patient that opened this chapter. Put simply, you can take advantage of the limitations of various remote mediums to use pauses well, ask for clarification, focus on essential questions, and listen for all you are worth.

As obvious as it sounds, your patients will convey much more information than is contained in the words themselves. These are the cues that would not be contained in a transcript of the conversation. Attend to *how* they say what they say, and then reflect what you hear. For example:

- "I hear in your voice that you're not too enthusiastic about doing that."
- "You're feeling pretty discouraged at this point."
- "You sound hesitant about that."
- "You really like that idea!"

It's also fine to inquire about the meaning of what you hear. You don't have to specify the cues to which you're responding.

- "You grew silent just now. What are you experiencing?"
- "Let me check on something here. I wonder whether you're feeling anxious about this."
- "As you consider making this change, what are you thinking and feeling at this point?"
- "How comfortable are you with our conversation so far?"

Consider the challenges faced by this doctor we observed in practice, bending forward, looking at the floor to avoid distraction. He was talking on the phone to an elderly woman of 78 who wants him to fill out a form confirming his approval for her to continue driving her car. They are struggling to hear each other: she because she is hard of hearing, he because her accent is unfamiliar. She reports that her *only* social contact is driving twice a week an hour away to visit her son, disabled with spina bifida, who is in a care facility. The doctor looks up and notices in the onscreen records that she had had a fall several months ago. When he asks how the fall happened, she says, "I got dizzy at the top of the stairs and fell back down them." This doctor knew that while the more remote contact deprived him of the cues that normally lie at the heart of good practice, it was an invitation to be skillful and practice MI well. An agreed-upon decision on the telephone about the next step was there for both to feel satisfied with. The patient agreed to bring the forms down to the clinic if she came for a brief health check.

Conclusion

In sum, you can use MI effectively when a visit is not in person. Voice-only media can be sufficient; the addition of video contact may or may not increase the impact of a conversation about health-related change. Even when you cannot physically be with patients, they can hear your heart.

CHAPTER 16

MI for Health Care Administrators and Managers

The ear of the leader must ring with the voices of the people.

—WOODROW WILSON

Is MI relevant outside of the consulting room? If listening is important for the well-being and outcomes for patients, what about for those who serve them, whether they be clinicians, clerical staff, or whoever? Does MI offer administrators any guidance for improving their service? This chapter aims to address questions like these, knowing that readers can delve into this subject more thoroughly in Marshall and Nielson (2020).

Realizing the potential benefits of using MI in health care practice will be difficult under conditions that make patients feel passive and downhearted, or in an environment that has an impersonal and disempowering feel to it. Imagine this scenario, from the experience of one of us (SR):

"By the time I found the clinic below ground level, down countless corridors, I had already seen many sick people. At the counter called 'Reception' most of the window was taken up by the back of a computer, with wires all over the place. A head appeared and a voice asked, 'Name?' and then said, 'Take a seat please.' We sat in five rows of plastic chairs in a windowless waiting room. More than an hour later I heard my name called, and a friendly nurse ushered me into a room where he took my name, date of birth, blood pressure, and weight, and then ushered me back out into the waiting room.

Then half an hour later, another nurse, more waiting, and then the doctor was reading my chart as I came into her office. Everyone opened the consultation by asking me the same questions about my name and date of birth. I got out of there as fast as I could."

If the overriding experience of a patient in your clinic is one of having things done *to* or *on* them, rather than *with* or *for* them, it's hard to see how they will walk out feeling empowered, no matter how skilled the individual practitioner is with MI. In contrast, if patients feel welcome and connected with people who show they care for them and for each other, the impact of MI in the consultation takes hold, and patients do better.

This chapter looks at what it might take for a provider or agency to implement principles of MI institutionwide and, by so doing, improve its culture. We use that term "culture" in talking about the overall tone, attitude, feel, and values (implied and overt) of a health care organization. This could be a private practitioner's office, a community health agency, a physiotherapy provider, a college health center, a family clinic, a walk-in drug treatment facility, a hospital, an urgent care center, an emergency department, or any other service aiming to help people with health needs. The culture of places like these comprises the values, beliefs, expectations, and attitudes that run through them. These threads have an impact on what it's like to be a patient in such places, and on what it's like to be an employee there. Indeed, it turns out that the principles and practice of MI not only can improve the quality of the care you provide patients, but they can also serve your organization's leadership in getting the best from the staff they manage (see Marshall & Nielsen, 2020).

Health care settings have values, beliefs, expectations, and attitudes running through them.

Improving the Environment

The environment or *culture* of a clinic or other health care setting embraces many things, from the architecture and physical layout of an office with its notices and seating arrangements, and even furniture, right through to the people who work there, how they interact with patients and each other, and the procedures they develop. The environment also includes the approach to decision making and style of interactions of the administrators who set up and maintain the system. Can efficiency and a caring, empowering environment be synchronized? The principles of MI work toward reaching this very goal.

CONSIDER: A Clinician's Story

In day-to-day practice it felt that the patients were not the priority, and there was a greater focus on getting through waiting lists and following standards and protocols with a pressure to show improved outcomes. I did ask myself, "Is this really what I trained for?" Learning MI rooted me in a purpose that went beyond surviving the day, to helping my patients make the most of their time with me. I moved away from being the detective who solved problems to being the guide who helped patients to say what they wanted and how they might get there. I felt the strain lift from my shoulders and then enjoyed my job. Colleagues became interested in what was different for me, and I supported their development. Over time we observed improved engagement and less drop out from the patients we worked with. Bit by bit, our service culture improved. This shift in service culture was never imposed but grew from a place of genuine desire to be helpful.

—ORLA ADAMS, *dietitian*

If your organization intends to improve its culture and effectiveness, patient and staff well-being is a worthwhile starting point. Keep in mind that change takes time, and that no single adjustment is likely to have major impact. Improving the culture is not just a matter of being more friendly to patients; there are a host of other routes to improvement. Give some thought to these questions:

- How do patients experience the service or agency? Can the facility itself be made more welcoming? To start answering that, conversations with patients will initially be of greater value than surveys. Have you invited them to comment on wait times, on interaction with the staff, or even on the physical environment of your waiting room and offices?
- What about waiting lists and other procedures? Can they be adjusted to give patients a more welcoming feel, to speed things up, or even to give patients greater choice?
- Are the mission and values of your practice or institution clear to the whole staff? Can you invite staff to describe those values in their own words?
- Are the staff matched appropriately to their assigned roles? How do they feel about their work, and about their interactions with their supervisors and upper management? Caring conversations and listening will help you address these questions. Like patients, staff usually prefer to feel heard and take part in decision making.

- What do the staff already know (or assume) about patient engagement? What's the first thing they say to patients? Consider the power of a question like "What matters the most to you today?" (see Barry & Edgman-Levitan, 2012). You could ask that question of your staff as well.
- If routine assessment is used, how might it be carried out in a more engaging and collaborative way (see Chapter 13)?

In patient consultations as well as when working with staff, the key components of providing excellent service in the organization are caring conversations and skillful *listening*. Nurturing these components in your organization's staff should help to improve its culture.

Walking the Talk

Change in an organization usually comes best by involving staff in the journey, whether they are practitioners, technicians, cleaners, or clerical staff. For the administrator, there is much to be gained by "walking the talk," modeling good leadership by listening to the experiences of practitioners, support staff, and patients. Imposing change from the top down, by decree, will have limited impact—similar to what happens inside the consultation when a practitioner tells a patient how to change, and then is met with resistance. To make real improvements in the culture, the organization's employees need to be involved, their input sought and valued. Any conversation with practitioners and others in the organization that starts by asking how *they* would like to improve things starts to resemble the practice of MI. As in the consultation room, the logic of MI is not to solve problems or have all the answers, but to listen to the staff's concerns and aspirations. If they feel valued and safe, they often come up with creative ideas for change.

ADMINISTRATOR: I want to see how we can make the environment here work better all-round, so that staff find life easier and more enjoyable, and patients see us as a friendly supportive group who get things done. It is a big ask, but I wonder what you might suggest, knowing we will need patience as things improve.

EMPLOYEE: That would take 30 years! Only kidding, but thanks for asking. It is quite a difficult question.

ADMINISTRATOR: I wonder where you might start?

EMPLOYEE: The waiting room for me. I say that because it would not be difficult to change things. I mean, why do we have this ugly window here, and those rows of chairs?

ADMINISTRATOR: You can see a way to make the room more friendly, or is this also about efficiency for you?

EMPLOYEE: Well, for a start, it makes no sense to have people queuing up like this. It just makes us feel stressed, and then those rows of chairs are unfriendly. Last week a patient at the back of the queue blew up and started yelling, and I thought we had a full-blown bust-up around the corner.

ADMINISTRATOR: I heard about that. Tough situation, and you can see a way to make things better.

EMPLOYEE: Yes, well, could we . . . ? (*Explains how the environment might look and feel.*)

Seen in this light, an administrator can use the insights and skills of MI to get the best out of staff, for the benefit of patients. Service or agency improvement is best viewed not as an event, but as the phased and unfolding outcome of conversations with staff and patients. We came across one team who served young people with diabetes who must have had many conversations like that above. The outcome was this: On arrival, the young people were offered a choice about who they wanted to see on that day. The service had to handle fewer consultations, clients had less waiting time, and this closely knit team was able to troubleshoot patient problems more efficiently. Over time, both the provider service and patient outcomes improved, and the consultations were more satisfying and patient-led.

A thorough examination of what service improvement might involve, including how MI can assist leadership teams, is provided by Marshall and Nielson (2020). In the next section, we discuss how you can help your staff gain MI skills.

> **Use the skills of MI to get the best out of staff, for the benefit of patients.**

Learning MI

Who in the staff group might learn what aspect of MI? It could be argued that while the entire staff in a health care organization can benefit from adopting MI principles, those who provide the care might want to learn more. There is no one way to introduce MI into a service; rather, it is a series of choices. Here are a few general reminders that have served the test of time in our training efforts:

- MI is not for everyone. Take this into account wherever possible.
- MI is a style of conversation, not a technique used on people. This involves a mindset shift for many in your organization, well worth high-lighting as useful in itself, for the sake of their own well-being and that of their patients.

There is no one way to introduce MI into a service.

- People in different jobs, at different points in their careers, will vary in their learning needs and how they might use MI. A recep-tionist might make use of some elements, an administrator oth-ers. Clinicians' use will vary, too.
- When it comes to the clinicians, they do best to learn on the job, reflect about their practice, discuss scenarios with colleagues, and also take feedback. Formal time set aside for training workshop(s) works well against this background.
- A commonly asked question, "How long does it take to train people in MI?", is not easy to answer because clinicians vary in initial competence levels, the skills involved require changes that are subtle, and getting this right calls for ongoing practice.
- There are reliable instruments available for quality assurance in MI (Hurlocker, Madson, & Schumacher, 2020).

The Spirit of MI, Listening, and Connecting

The case for introducing everyone in a service to the spirit of MI is strengthened by the observation that almost everyone in the organiza-tion talks with patients and thus can have an impact on their well-being. The aim here would not be so much to teach how MI informs clinical practice as to explore with them the value of coming alongside and lis-tening to people, including colleagues, and of not jumping in too quickly with giving advice. The fundamental shift from directing to guiding often rings bells for people because they see its wider relevance outside of work, with relatives and friends.

For example, using the information and advice-giving skills of MI (see the framework in Chapter 11) will enrich the quality of even those informal brief conversations the staff have with each other and with patients. You can convey the essence of *offering*, in the spirit of MI, with just a few brief learning events.

In training clinicians in MI, it is best to employ a variety of meth-ods. Research on this topic suggests that workshops alone don't impact practice, especially if delivered as one-off events. The MI research on this subject points to the following guidelines (see the Appendix, "Devel-oping MI Skillfullness"):

- Give people a solid overview of what MI is and how it sounds in practice. A tell–show–try mixture works well, first explaining, then demonstrating, and finally practicing component skills.
- Like many medical and nursing skills, observed practice with feedback is what improves competence over time.
- Learning MI is not an event but a process. Be patient with your team, and advise them to be patient with themselves. Skillfulness can continue to develop throughout one's career.
- Perhaps the best indicator of good MI practice is how patients respond to it. Investigate ways of gauging your patient's experiences with your agency. (Fidelity in delivering MI predicts positive outcomes for patients; Miller & Rollnick, 2014.)

If formal MI training is not an option, an alternative approach, illustrated in the dietician's story previously, would be to encourage just a few practitioners to become proficient in MI. This allows for a more organic and phased integration of MI. We worked with one manager of a large inner-city hospital respiratory medicine service who organized lunchtime get-togethers for the whole team to discuss MI and new learning opportunities.

Almost everyone in the organization talks with patients and thus can have an impact on their well-being.

MI in Public Health Settings

There is encouraging evidence that MI can impact the lives of people from disadvantaged backgrounds (Hettema, Steele, & Miller, 2005). Unfortunately, however, most of these patients receive care in a suboptimal environment, leaving administrators facing a paradox that is hard to avoid, originally called the "inverse care law" (Hart, 1971): Patients and services in the greatest need for quality care are least likely to get it. Can MI gain traction under these circumstances, such as in underresourced community health centers, where practitioners are often less well paid and more likely to be weighed down by shorter consultation times and a heavier burden all around; where managers themselves are also taking strain? One answer seems to be in the potential of MI to relieve pressure on practitioners.

CONSIDER: Does Using MI Reduce Stress and Burnout?

In marginalized communities we discovered that practitioners in public health feel increasingly obliged to make patients address their lifestyle, telling them to do this, do that, and that this was in itself causing practitioners stress and affecting their own wellbeing. Our use of MI in training efforts, both online and in person, therefore started with their wellbeing and how they might take that weight off their shoulders to solve every problem they come across. Then we helped them with a few key adjustments to using a guiding style in their everyday practice. One key lesson was that support from management was critical.

—GOODMAN SIBEKO, MD, PhD

Conclusion

How can you improve the experience your patients have with your organization? Putting patients first has to be more than a catch phrase or a note on a poster in the break room. Basic MI principles can make the culture of your service more collaborative, respectful, and responsive to patients, leading to better health outcomes. MI skills used in clinical practice can make interventions more impactful. How can you make this happen in your office? Start the conversations with all involved, to show them you care, to ask them how something like MI might be of help, and to develop clarity about why and how this might come about. Establishing MI in a health care setting is a bit like planting a flower. It takes time and patience, and evidence suggests that good patient outcomes are there for the taking.

INSIDE MOTIVATIONAL INTERVIEWING

In Part V, we take a look inside the consultation, with two in-depth examples. It is here, observing the flow of a conversation, that you can make the most progress in learning MI.

We start with a scenario in Chapter 17 that involves continuity of care, where the practitioner can work with a patient over a number of consultations. In this case, the challenge is how to help a woman gain greater confidence in a vaccine for her child. In Chapter 18, we use the example of a consultation with a hostile patient, and challenge you at various junctions, where we ask you how you might respond (and we offer some of our own ideas, too).

CHAPTER 17

Vaccine Hesitancy

A Case Example

The best response to a lie is not a fact
but a deeper truth.

— JON LOVETT

It's a routine clinic, and when Maria, the practitioner, raises the subject of a child's vaccination for measles she is taken aback by the mother's response. Maria knew she had to be prepared for the unexpected, but this felt like an altogether higher level, where the mother replied with a torrent of misinformation and resistance to the idea of vaccination. The temptation was there to reach out for the righting reflex and correct the mother's misunderstanding. Even if Maria is well versed in using MI, she can't necessarily avoid that visceral experience of shock, followed by the desire to put things to right.

For the mother, Helen, she neither needed nor wanted correcting and fixing. She was busy enough and couldn't wait to get out of the clinic. As Dick Cavett said, "It's a rare person who wants to hear what she doesn't want to hear." So, what now for Maria and Helen?

We use a case example here (and in Chapter 18) as a way of integrating what we have covered in the previous chapters, to give you a feel for how all of the parts of the book fit together: the spirit, the skills, and the four processes. Even if you don't ever talk with patients about vaccines, you will recognize the familiar challenges: holding back, coming alongside, drawing out the solutions and decisions from them. Our goal is to show how the use of MI can run right

Using MI in a consultation can make a difference to your well-being and the patient's.

through a consultation, mistakes and all, and make a difference to your well-being, the patient's well-being, and the clinical outcome, too.

People who feel hesitant about a vaccine are not usually as initially dogmatic or resistant as Helen is in this scenario. More often they are feeling ambivalent, worried about side effects and other issues. However, we chose this example because it allows us to highlight how MI can be used in difficult consultations.

The exchange below is split across three conversations, mainly to help us illustrate different aspects of MI, and because in many clinic settings one does have time for short conversations spread over time.

First Conversation

The consultation started well, despite one mistake that Maria made.

Engaging and Providing Focus

MARIA: While you are here, Helen, with this little boy just over a year old now, it's time to think about the vaccine called MMR, for measles, mumps, and rubella.

HELEN: That one, no thanks. That causes autism, not for us, thanks. You think I would put poison into my child? The drug company no doubt makes millions off of us, and I am their guinea pig? No thanks. Can I go now?

COMMENT

A reaction as strong as this signals the need to *only engage*, to "sit on your hands," hold back from fixing a problem and adjust one's mindset from that of a fixer to a compassionate and curious guide. Noticing your emotional reaction and responding wisely is a crucial reflective skill when using MI. "Take a step back and listen" is what Maria said to herself.

Only Engaging

MARIA: That's a strong reaction! How do you see this MMR vaccine?

HELEN: As I say, this is really not for us. You should hear the stories I have heard. No offense to you, you are just doing your job but I don't trust those drug companies and the power they have.

Just in it for the money if you ask me. Not for my little boy. I won't put poison in his blood.

MARIA: Well, yes, I *am* just doing my job here, and I have no wish to oblige you to take anything you don't want to. [*Emphasizing autonomy*]

HELEN: I know that. I usually look forward to coming down here.

MARIA: It's your child and his precious little body, and you're determined to make decisions that are best for him. [*Listening statement*]

HELEN: Yes, that's right. When I first heard about this from other moms like me, I was shocked. I mean they just went along with it knowing about these stories about autism, as if that's a risk they would take.

MARIA: What exactly have you heard about this MMR vaccine?

HELEN: I heard about children who became autistic after getting the vaccine, and there have been senior doctors who have advised against it.

MARIA: Would you like me to give you a leaflet so you can think about it all?

HELEN: Thanks, definitely not.

MARIA: Maybe when I see you next time, we can chat about this again, okay? You won't be offended?

HELEN: Not at all.

COMMENT

The conversation went fine until Maria offered the leaflet. Then the door was firmly shut. Why? Here are some possibilities:

1. Maria stopped engaging and jumped ahead to solution talk.
2. Maria used the righting reflex and the patient backed off.
3. Maria wanted to end the consultation, and this was a reasonable way of doing it.

Maria's investment in a minute of engaging was not wasted when she made this small mistake. If you are genuine, accepting, and compassionate, the patient usually won't mind. Resisting the impulse to correct, and

Resisting the impulse to correct is an investment in itself.

listening instead, is an investment in itself. What would Helen have said about that conversation? Maybe something like this: "Maria is okay, she wants the best for me, and at least she listened to me. I was glad to get out of there, though. That vaccine is not my top priority right now."

Second Conversation

At their next meeting a few weeks later, Maria knew not to dive straight in with a question like "How do feel now about the benefits of this MMR vaccine?" It's too early to ask an evoking question before engaging Helen first. Not only was she talking across a cultural divide (she was Hispanic, Helen was African American), but she also knew that just because you think you know and like a patient, it always helps to reengage at the next meeting. People's circumstances, mood, and attitude might have changed, as indeed was the case here.

Helen had been chatting to some other new mothers, and one of them used the words "fake news" to describe the anti–MMR vaccination movement. Helen wasn't convinced by that comment, but it did sow a little seed of doubt in her mind about the dangers of vaccines. Then she forgot about it and got on with life. At her next check-up, Maria was ready to reengage. The best route here was via a topic that united them both: the well-being of the child.

Focusing

MARIA: (*They talk for a while about the child's milestones and challenges with sleep.*) You might be angry with me now (*laughs*), but I wonder about that vaccine we talked about last time.

HELEN: No, I'm not angry, but I don't like all the pressure around this.

MARIA: So, if I don't put pressure on you, you might not mind chatting about this. [*Listening statement*]

HELEN: Well, I haven't made my mind up and I don't plan to rush into this right now.

MARIA: And, that's your choice. Would you prefer to leave this to another time? It's fine by me if that's what you want. [*Emphasizing autonomy*]

HELEN: No, it's okay. What would you like to say?

MARIA: Mainly that this is completely your decision, and that I have some information I would like to share with you. Then, it's your call.

HELEN: Go ahead then.

COMMENT

Has Maria been transparent about her role and what her view is? Has she put pressure on Helen to accept her view? Probably "yes" to the first question and "no" to the second. It helps to cement trust by being open and at the same time championing choice for the patient.

> MARIA: The best way to start is probably here. What do you understand about this vaccine? Then I can see whether there is information you might find useful. How do you see it? [*Ask*]
>
> HELEN: Well, I'm not a doctor or anything, but you put this stuff into a kid and then what? Some of them get serious side effects. How do I know what the truth is?
>
> MARIA: You have heard conflicting messages and you are not sure what to believe. [*Listening statement*]
>
> HELEN: I heard that some doctors have warned against this vaccine, so this is not easy for me.
>
> MARIA: . . . Because you want to make the best decision for your little boy. [*Listening statement*]
>
> HELEN: Of course, I do, so I don't need pressure from you people down here to be honest.
>
> MARIA: I don't mean to put pressure on you. I just want to give you the facts.
>
> HELEN: I just don't believe your leaflets and things.

COMMENT

What's happened now? Maria wondered whether she had made a mistake by saying, "I just want to give you the facts." She had started using the righting reflex to correct Helen's understanding. So, Helen backed away. Yet there is a way to proceed by *offering* information that empowers not corrects a patient.

> MARIA: You want to make your own mind up, without pressure, in your own time. [*Listening statement*]
>
> HELEN: Exactly.
>
> MARIA: May I offer you some information to see what you make of it?

HELEN: Sure, I know that you want the best for my boy.

MARIA: We are both united there. That's why I do this job, to see smiling babies and happy mothers. (*They both laugh.*) Here's the puzzle, see what you make of it. [*Offer*] The researcher who suggested a link with autism has since been censured for research that was not accurate. So, it's no wonder that people in your situation feel confused about this because misinformation can spread like a virus, a bit like the way a rumor spreads. What do you think? [*Ask*]

HELEN: Yeah, that's what I heard. A friend of mine said, "Don't take it," and then someone else said people were spreading misinformation about the link with autism.

MARIA: It's hard to know who to trust. [*Listening statement*]

HELEN: Yeah, that's right.

MARIA: And then, there might be other concerns you have. I wonder what else might help you with this decision? [*Ask*]

HELEN: What are the side effects that you notice here in the clinic?

MARIA: (*Goes through a few of the most common side effects and mentions the much less common ones, too.*) So, that's quite a lot from my side. I wonder how helpful that was? [*Ask*]

HELEN: Yeah, it is a lot to take in. I think I'll discuss this with my boyfriend and my best friend, okay?

MARIA: You are carefully weighing things and want to make a decision that's right for you. [*Affirmation and listening statement that emphasizes autonomy*]

HELEN: Yes, that's right.

COMMENT

The more Maria held back from expressing her views or putting pressure on Helen, the freer Helen felt to open up and consider change. Offering information like this is a skill set likely to have considerable impact on change, whether this be in lifestyle, adherence, or some other area. Maria also conveyed much of the spirit of MI (see Chapter 1): She communicated that both she and the mother are in *partnership* for the health of Helen's child, expressed *compassionate* concern for the boy's well-being, *empowered* Helen to make her own decisions, *accepted* her reservations as legitimate concern for her son. Maria used a good range of core skills, too.

Third Conversation

There was disappointment for Maria when she raised the subject again during this third conversation. Was Helen ever going to make up her mind? Nothing had changed. Maria decided to engage briefly and then to approach Helen's ambivalence using the simple idea of letting her weigh the pros and cons.

> HELEN: I knew you were going to ask me again, and sorry, I can't make up my mind.
>
> MARIA: Are you okay to talk this over for a few minutes?
>
> HELEN: Sure, I do trust you, Maria.
>
> MARIA: What's the hesitation about for you?
>
> HELEN: I don't want my boy to get measles [*Change talk*], but it's the side effects that still worry me. [*Sustain talk*]
>
> MARIA: So, you're aware that measles can be serious. [*Listening statement*] Is it the autism thing that still bothers you, or are you worried about other side effects?
>
> HELEN: Well, my boyfriend is more laid-back and happy to go with the vaccine, and I am more cautious. But, that autism thing sounds like a hoax.
>
> MARIA: You are not as concerned as you were about autism, but you still have this worry about side effects. [*Listening statement*]
>
> HELEN: That's right.
>
> MARIA: Is there anything about the vaccine I can help you with by way of information and that kind of thing?
>
> HELEN: No, not really.

COMMENT

On the platform of the engagement she had established, Maria turned to helping Helen to clarify for herself the pros and cons of taking the vaccine.

> MARIA: Why don't you go through in your own mind how you see the pros and cons, and I'll just listen. It often helps people to see things a bit more clearly. Would that be okay?
>
> HELEN: Sure.
>
> MARIA: Let's look at the downside of this vaccine. How do you really see this right now?

HELEN: Okay, well, I now feel less concerned about that autism idea, and me and my boyfriend reckon it could be like fake news and that sort of thing, so I don't trust that as much as I did. But, I am still worried about this being like putting a foreign substance into my little boy that gives him side effects and makes him not well. [*Sustain talk*]

COMMENT

Maria felt the immediate sting of hearing misinformation here with that reference to "a foreign substance," knowing that Helen did not really understand what the vaccine contains and how it works. However, since she had initiated this exploration of pros and cons, she made a conscious decision to let Helen continue.

MARIA: I get you. It's hard to see how this might actually be good for him, even though you have heard it can prevent him from getting a serious illness like measles. [*Listening statement*]

HELEN: Yes, that's how I feel.

MARIA: And, what about the benefits of the vaccine?

HELEN: Well, I sat down with my boyfriend and we looked at what happens with measles on the Internet, and it opened our eyes. This is a nasty illness, that's for sure. I also never knew that the more people get vaccinated, the more it kills the bug in the community. So, we kind of said, maybe we should go for this. [*Change talk*]

MARIA: You are united in doing the right thing for your boy [*Affirmation*], and you don't want him to catch this measles bug. [*Listening statement*]

HELEN: We are beginning to find information that we trust, which helps as well.

MARIA: So, you have this background worry about side effects and also you know you don't want him to get measles. [*Listening statement*]

HELEN: That about sums it up.

MARIA: What do you think is best?

HELEN: I'm going to call my boyfriend when I leave this place, and if he agrees, we may go for it, I think. [*Change talk*] I'm still nervous about it, if you know what I mean. [*Sustain talk*]

MARIA: You are going to connect with him first, and then you trust that the two of you will make the right decision. [*Listening statement*]

HELEN: Yes, and if we decide to go for it, can I bring him back?

MARIA: My schedule is okay this morning, so just come right back and tell reception you are here, all right?

That question, "What do you think is best?", is an excellent outcome of examining ambivalence. It is the patient's choice. All Maria did was ask Helen about the pros and cons and step aside and listen as she weighed them. You will notice that her listening statements were very crisp, and she made sincere efforts to reflect back what she understood Helen to be saying and feeling. It took just a minute or two, and it was notable also for the way Maria did not step in with pointed questions, let alone change the subject or divert the conversation toward providing information or advice. The less she pushed or urged Helen, the more progress was made.

There's an ongoing discussion in and beyond the field of MI about to what extent you should consciously steer the conversation in favor of change. After all, Maria could easily have asked more open questions about the benefits of vaccination, and reinforced Helen's change talk by using further listening statements. On this occasion, she did not have lots of time and chose instead to invest her energy in capturing the essence of how Helen felt, to very good effect. The rudder that steered that exchange was Helen's own sense of what was best.

Sometimes, simply looking at the pros and cons, without steering the conversation in the direction of change, can reinforce rather than help someone to resolve ambivalence (Miller & Rose, 2015). Whether you steer the conversation gently in the direction of change depends on the problem being discussed, your judgment about what is in the patient's best interest, and what they say they want.

> Simply looking at the pros and cons can reinforce rather than help to resolve ambivalence.

In this last chapter on practical applications of MI, it has been fitting to raise this quite complex issue. Making these judgments requires a degree of skill and thoughtfulness that is worth pursuing, bearing in mind that the alternative, simply correcting or persuading someone to change, is more often than not an abrasive experience that undermines patient choice. It is possible to be transparent about your view about change, as Maria did above in a number of ways. The rest was left up to Helen to decide.

Conclusion

Looking back at this exchange between Maria and Helen, and indeed at earlier chapters, too, we are struck by how a potentially complex conversation can be made easier by not trying to be clever. Rather, if you free up your mind of clutter and ambition for the patient, it's a simple matter of handing over the resolution to them, aided by offering, not imposing, information and advice and by highlighting change talk as it emerges. This evoking process is a pleasure and a privilege to participate in. As patients hear themselves speak and weigh alternatives, a clearer perspective emerges along with sometimes brave and life-changing decisions.

CHAPTER 18

MI in Depth
"What Would You Say Next?"

Love and compassion are necessities, not luxuries.
Without them humanity cannot survive.
—The Dalai Lama

Using an illustrative patient interview, this last chapter offers two things. First, we take a look inside the decisions one makes when using MI in tough circumstances with a hostile patient. Then second, at key junctions in the conversation, we invite you to consider how you might respond to the patient and we also offer some of our own ideas. (You can view a dramatization of this consultation on YouTube. It's titled "Motivational Interviewing in Brief Consultations," and you can find it with the search terms "Rollnick, BMJ.")

Though the interview used in this chapter is not perfect (no consultation ever is), it contains almost all the characteristics of MI and associated skills described earlier in the book. We pay attention at the outset to the practitioner's state of mind as a key driver of good practice in MI.

The Brief

An overweight patient, Mr. Smith was to be given medication for hypertension, and the practitioner needed to raise the subject of his weight. The detailed brief stated:

Mr. Smith is a 60-year-old man who has come to see his GP [general practitioner] for a medication review. He takes verapamil (160 mg three times a day) and ramipril (5 mg once daily). His blood pressure is currently 138/88 mm Hg. He weighs 110 kg [about 242.5 pounds] and is 172.2 cm [about 5 feet, 7 inches] tall, with a BMI [body mass index] of around 37. The GP wants to raise the subject of weight, and soon realizes that Mr. Smith is angry and that the consultation could become difficult to manage if not handled carefully.

Whom Are You Meeting?

Is this just another patient with a list of problems or a person with strengths as well? What you say to the patient will be influenced by how

> **What you say to the patient will be influenced by how you view them. Avoid focusing strictly on their problems.**

you view them. The trap to avoid here is being pulled into the mindset of a deficit detective (Chapter 1, page 12), only interested in problems and their resolution. Mr. Smith is a person first, patient second. You will want to empathize, notice strengths, and work with those strengths.

But, He Is Hostile

Imagine you are about to see a hostile Mr. Smith. Chances are that your heart sinks, and you think, "Oh no, this won't be easy." Is your equilibrium upset by anticipating this anger and are you wondering how you might defend yourself?

Now consider a different view: it might not be helpful to label him a difficult patient in the first place. There might be good reason why he is so upset. If you are practicing MI, instead of working against him by defending yourself or the clinic staff, you come alongside. This was the approach taken here—*not* to argue back or defend oneself, but to respond by listening, on the grounds that unless someone feels heard they are unlikely to collaborate in the consultation.

We will step back from the consultation in four places below to consider how you might respond. There is no single best way to proceed. Anticipating how the patient might respond to what you say is a skill

> **Maintain the spirit of MI: What you say is guided by curiosity and compassion.**

well worth practicing. Above all, you need to maintain the spirit of MI, whereby what you say is guided by curiosity and compassion, with a keen eye on how the patient might lead a healthy life.

The Consultation

> PRACTITIONER: Well Mr. Smith, that's your medication sorted out. Blood pressure is a little on the high side. I wonder if I could raise the subject of your weight.
>
> MR. SMITH: What?
>
> PRACTITIONER: I wondered if we could spend just a couple of minutes talking about your weight.
>
> MR. SMITH: You are joking aren't you?! I mean, look—I've made time in my day to come here. I'm kept in your waiting room for 45 minutes, it's not acceptable. You know? If I make an appointment with a client for 10, I expect it to start at 10, not quarter to 11.

> **STOP!** Before you read on, consider what you would say next and why you would say that.
>
> Your reply: _____

Here are three different possible responses from us, all of them consistent with MI:

> WILLIAM R. MILLER: "You're really furious about having to wait so long." I might reflect the angry feeling that he is expressing so that he knows I hear him.
>
> CHRISTOPHER C. BUTLER: "I know what you mean. I hate keeping people waiting, and I am sorry about what has happened. The pressure we are all under is horrendous, and emergencies can set back the whole day. I am sure your world can be just as tough." This depersonalizes the problem, de-escalates the tension, and suggests common experience and purpose, such that, in a way, "we are all in this together."
>
> STEPHEN ROLLNICK: "It's been really frustrating today to be kept waiting like that." That is a simple listening statement, one way of expressing empathy for Mr Smith.

What actually happened was that the practitioner offered a series of listening statements:

> PRACTITIONER: Right. And so you're busy enough, and . . . [*Listening statement*]

MR. SMITH: Yeah, I've got other things to do. I've got accounts to do, I've got clients that are coming in, you know?

PRACTITIONER: And, it wasn't necessarily easy for you to make the time to come down, and you had to wait in the waiting room, and now I raise the subject of weight with you. [*Listening statement*]

MR. SMITH: I mean yeah, okay, fair enough. I've got to have my blood pressure medication changed, but I really haven't got time to talk about my weight. I mean, you know, I'm aware of my weight, I'm aware of the problems, and also I'm aware of the solutions. [*Change talk*] So, I don't really need a discussion. It's just that I've got too much to do.

PRACTITIONER: Right, and so it's been a bit of a rush for you coming in. [*Listening statement*]

MR. SMITH: Yeah.

PRACTITIONER: And, I am sorry about the wait in the waiting room.

MR. SMITH: Well, it's bad form you know?

PRACTITIONER: Yeah, and that's not easy for you because you'd like to go really soon, and here I am asking you to spend just a couple of minutes with me.

MR. SMITH: Yeah, basically I've got things to do, I've got to get back to the office, I've got a pile of work that I've got to deal with, and every moment out of my day means I have to work in the evening or weekends.

PRACTITIONER: It counts. [*Listening statement*]

MR. SMITH: Well, when you're self-employed, you haven't got a choice, you know?

STOP!	Before you read on, consider what you would say next and why you would say that.

Your reply: _____

Again, there are various MI-consistent ways you could respond here:

WILLIAM R. MILLER: "I do apologize for the wait. You're a busy man." An apology is one way to respond to discord like this, acknowledging the inconvenience and accepting partial responsibility for it, then following it with a reflective listening statement.

CHRISTOPHER C. BUTLER: "That said, since we are both wanting you to get the most out of this consultation and, ultimately, for you to be as healthy as possible, a few minutes together on this could be useful." This response identifies a collaborative common purpose, with the patient's interests, rather than the medical agenda, driving the process.

STEPHEN ROLLNICK: "I wonder what this means for you right now? It's really your call whether we have a chat now or not." This hands responsibility over to Mr. Smith. It is a bit of a high-risk statement because he might say "no" to the discussion, but to me that would also be acceptable.

What actually happened next was the practitioner emphasizing personal choice:

PRACTITIONER: Exactly. It's up to you. Just a couple of minutes?

MR. SMITH: Well . . . I'm here now. So yeah, okay, if it's just a couple of minutes.

PRACTITIONER: I promise.

MR. SMITH: Okay, because I really must get on.

PRACTITIONER: I want to simply ask you how you feel about it? [*Open question*]

MR. SMITH: About what? Losing weight? Well, obviously I want to. Umm, yeah, I mean who doesn't? I mean, I'm aware I'm over my balanced weight, and I know that it's causing problems. I mean obviously I get out of breath if I have to do something a bit strenuous, and I realize that I'm on this blood pressure medicine, and I realize that's probably contributing to it. [*Change talk*]

STOP!	Before you read on, consider what you would say next and why you would say that.
Your reply: _____	

Here are three different ideas from the authors:

WILLIAM R. MILLER: "You're a man who's honest about what's happening." I might offer an affirmation at this point that he does see the link between his weight and health. Phrasing it in this way makes it a complex affirmation about the kind of person he is.

CHRISTOPHER C. BUTLER: "For sure! It sounds like you are fully up to speed, as you say, about your weight situation and the potential benefits to you if you were able to shed a few pounds then." This affirmation, summary, and reflective statement might invite some change talk from the patients about benefits to them from taking a crack at attempting weight loss. I would be surprised if some self-motivating statements did not follow.

STEPHEN ROLLNICK: "You are juggling a lot at the moment, with work demands especially, and a balanced weight is not necessarily easy for you to maintain." I picked up this idea of balance and juggling in his life as a whole and made a listening statement that also captured how he might be feeling about his weight.

What happened next was the practitioner offered a complex reflection:

PRACTITIONER: You can see the links between your weight and your health. And, you'd like things to be a bit better. [*Listening statement*]

MR. SMITH: I mean yeah, there are other things, but yeah the weight is something I would like to get hold of. [*Change talk*]

PRACTITIONER: You'd like to if you could. [*Listening statement*]

MR. SMITH: Yeah, I know the theories—a bit of exercise on a regular basis, a balanced diet. [*Change talk*] But unfortunately, because of my lifestyle, because of being a self-employed accountant, it's finding the time to exercise, but also finding the time to think, "Okay, I'm going to go shopping for this, that, and the other," prepare a meal . . . [*Sustain talk*] with me it's very often . . .

PRACTITIONER: Ready meals and that sort of thing.

MR. SMITH: Yeah, food on the run, you know. Grazing.

STOP! Before you read on, consider what you would say next and why you would say that.

Your reply: _____

One more time, here are three possible responses from the authors:

WILLIAM R. MILLER: "That's quite a challenge. How might you be able to fit some healthier eating into your hectic daily schedule?" A temptation here is to give some advice, but instead I would ask him for his own suggestions.

CHRISTOPHER C. BUTLER: "You have obviously given this some thought then about how you might make progress." This affirms the patient as an engaged problem-solver, and invites them to mention one or two positive steps they could identify that might work for them.

STEPHEN ROLLNICK: "Yet getting hold of your weight is quite a high priority for you." "Getting hold of" is a phrase he used, and I remembered this. I wanted to highlight the change talk I had heard.

What actually happened next was the practitioner offered a summary:

PRACTITIONER: Let me see if I can summarize what you've said. And, then we'll see what's next. You lead a busy life. You run a business, and you've got a lot to do. You're aware of the links between your health and your weight, and you are concerned to some extent about them. And ideally, it sounds like, you would like to do something about it. It's just that your life is busy and rushed, and you tend to use convenience foods in order to get the work done. [*Summary*]

MR. SMITH: Yeah, to a certain extent because of my lifestyle, food is just fuel because I'm juggling all of these balls and I don't want to drop them.

PRACTITIONER: Okay. And so if you could fit it in, you would like things to be different, but that's not so easy. [*Listening statement*] Can I suggest that you come back and see me in a couple of weeks' time? Just to chat about this.

MR. SMITH: Umm, okay, I'm up for that, but it's going to be the same problem. A, finding time, and B, if I make an appointment, I don't expect to be kept waiting for half an hour.

PRACTITIONER: Exactly. I tell you what might be a nice solution: if you come down for the first appointment, and I give you an appointment at 8:30. Then, there will be absolutely no waiting. The purpose of that visit will be to have a look at how you really feel about how you could move forward, and somehow fit a healthier lifestyle into the busy work life that you've got.

MR. SMITH: I'll maybe have a look at my schedule, see whether anything can be arranged, or I can pass something on to someone, so it's not a wasted interview. So, I can come here and say I've looked at my schedule, I've looked into things . . . whatever. [*Change talk*]

PRACTITIONER: Good. And, see if you can fix it up but also give some thought to what we've talked about.

MR. SMITH: Yeah, of course. Sorry I went off a bit.

Evident in each of the four stopping-off points above is that there is not just one correct response to what a patient says. Yet, what you say clearly matters and impacts the direction of the conversation that follows. That distinction between the eagle and the mouse seems relevant here (see Chapter 8, page 80): At the level of the mouse, where you respond moment-to-moment to what's in front of you, it pays to imagine how the patient might respond before you ask a question or make a listening statement. Then, at the level of the eagle, where you are looking ahead and can see the big picture, it helps to be guided by the spirit of MI: curious, compassionate, and in tricky situations like that above, always ready to use listening statements and to emphasise freedom of choice for the patient.

In that consultation, we saw all of the four processes (engage, focus, evoke, and plan), and the practitioner managed to achieve several important outcomes. The patient, Mr. Smith, left feeling heard and respected, and evidently was more engaged in working with the practitioner on his health. The ground is prepared now for sowing the seeds of a longer, more productive relationship in which the practitioner and Mr. Smith can work collaboratively.

> **Imagine how the patient might respond before you ask a question or make a listening statement.**

Conclusion

One of our most useful insights as we developed our MI skills was about the value of not cutting across or interrupting what the patient is saying, but rather acknowledging their perspective and only very gently nudging them in the direction of a healthier solution. This is less about being clever and more about keeping a keen and compassionate eye on what might be in their best interests.

When we started this work on MI in the early 1980s, we were soon made aware of its relevance in health care. Our focus at that time was on the motivation to change of the patient. Looking back, there was one omission, worth highlighting in the closing lines of this book: the well-being, mindset, and motivational state of the practitioner. Our hope now is that using MI takes pressure off you and that its use not only saves you time as your skills improve but also that patients notice this and respond well to the trust you bestow on them.

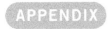

A Practitioner's Guide to MI Research

Clinical research on MI has grown rapidly in the 21st century. As we complete this book, there are over 1,600 controlled clinical trials in the literature and at least 140 systematic reviews and meta-analyses of MI research (e.g., Frost et al., 2016, 2018; Lundahl & Burke, 2009; McKenzie, Pierce, & Gunn, 2015; Thompson et al., 2011). To date, the largest meta-analysis focusing exclusively on MI encompassed only 119 clinical trials (Lundahl, Kunz, Brownell, Tollefson, & Burke, 2010). Understandably, most reviews now address specific subsets of this literature. We begin with some broad observations from clinical MI research, then proceed to discuss more specific applications of MI in health care relying primarily on systematic reviews and meta-analyses rather than individual clinical trials.

Reliable Findings from MI Research

Purpose of MI

Some health problems can be treated well with acute care medicine—infections and broken bones, for example. Other conditions can be caused and (ideally) resolved by changing health behaviors such as smoking and drinking, physical activity, healthy or unhealthy eating. Telling patients what to do can prompt a small proportion to make changes, but most people with chronic health problems are not doing what they need to do to be healthy. So, what can you do when what needs to change is a patient's behavior or lifestyle?

To oversimplify, MI is basically useful to help patients increase healthy behavior and decrease risky behavior. It is something you can do within the time confines of ordinary practice (Bischof, Bischof, & Rumpf, 2021). If you only have a short time and what is most needed is health behavior change, MI is a good choice and quite different from warning or scolding. It is not something to do instead of or in addition to routine care. It is a *way* of doing what you already do.

Overall Impact of MI

When delivered well, the average impact of MI is a small to medium effect on patients' behavior at home. Most clinical trials have tested outcomes from one or two MI visits ranging from 10 to 50 minutes. Trials generally support the efficacy of MI as compared to no additional intervention or brief advice. When MI is compared with other active interventions of greater intensity or duration, outcome differences tend to be minimal if any. Meta-analyses suggest that MI is somewhat more impactful when offered in more than one visit, and that it's worth spending a bit longer with patients when you can (Rubak, Sandbaek, Lauritzen, & Christensen, 2005). This can be valuable when you see the same patients over time.

What must also be said is that the effectiveness of MI is highly *variable*. A quarter to a third of clinical trials of MI have found no benefit. In multisite trials, MI works at some sites and not others (which happens with medications as well). There are also large outcome differences among providers, even within a clinical trial where the MI is more structured and closely monitored. Some practitioners just seem to be better at it, and the provider differences in outcome have to do, in part, with skillfulness in the practice of MI (Miller & Rollnick, 2014).

Developing MI Skillfulness

At first, we assumed that people would develop competence in MI just by coming to a training workshop. Not so. Participants' workshop evaluations were glowing, but when we compared audio recordings of clinical practice before and after training, very little evidence existed that we had been there (Miller & Mount, 2001). Worse still, the workshop participants believed that they *had* learned MI and were now using it proficiently in practice, so they saw little reason to learn more. There were a few prodigies who actually were delivering MI rather well after initial training, but on average the training had no significant effect on practice, certainly not enough to make any difference in patients' outcomes.

Thus began the quest for what it *does* take to develop competence in MI. There are now dozens of studies on MI training, enough to warrant systematic and meta-analytic reviews (Barwick, Bennett, Johnson, McGowan, & Moore, 2012; de Roten, Zimmerman, Ortega, & Despland, 2013; Dunhill, Schmidt, & Klein, 2014; Hall, Staiger, Simpson, Best, & Lubman, 2016; Kaczmarek, Kavanaugh, Lazzarini, Warnock, & Van Netten, in press; Keeley, Engel, Reed, Brody, & Burke, 2018; Schwalbe, Oh, & Zweben, 2014; Soderlund, Madson, Rubak, & Nilsen, 2011). When trained in MI, medical students can reach at least beginning levels of proficiency (Kaltman & Tankersley, 2020). It turns out that learning MI is rather like developing proficiency in any complex skill such as playing a sport or flying an airplane. You don't just read books, watch videos, or attend classroom training. What makes a difference is getting feedback and coaching from someone who observes you practicing. In one randomized trial of training strategies, we found that five 30-minute telephone coaching sessions were enough to substantially improve proficiency (Miller, Yahne, Moyers, Martinez, & Pirritano, 2004). A more recent study found that it took between 4 and 20 group coaching sessions to bring trainees up to a competence benchmark in MI (Schumacher et al., 2018). A key, then, seems to be *observed* practice with some feedback and coaching, which is how many medical procedures are learned.

Broad Applicability of MI

MI can be practiced effectively by a broad range of providers including physicians, nurses, dentists, behavioral health specialists, dieticians, health coaches, and diabetes educators. As will be apparent in what follows, MI has shown beneficial patient outcomes across a wide range of health conditions. It seems to cross cultures well (Bahafzallah, Hayden, Bouchal, Singh, & King-Shier, 2020), and is being taught and practiced in at least 61 languages around the world. Though MI was first developed to work with people who overuse alcohol, the basic method applies well across a broad range of clinical situations.

How Does MI Work?

There is now extensive research on the therapeutic mechanisms by which MI triggers behavior change, again enough to prompt reviews and meta-analyses (Apodaca & Longabaugh, 2009; Copeland, McNamara, Kelson, & Simpson, 2015; Magill et al., 2014, 2018, 2019; Pace et al., 2017; Romano & Peters, 2015, 2016). It is clear that what patients *say* during MI sessions matters. The ratio of client change talk to sustain talk is usually a better predictor of behavioral outcome than is either of these alone. Furthermore, the amount of change talk and sustain talk that patients express is clearly related to MI practitioner skill. Greater clinician MI skillfulness and higher rates of MI-consistent responses are linked to more patient change talk and less sustain talk. MI-inconsistent responses, on the other hand, evoke more patient sustain talk and worse outcomes. The causal link of clinician responses with patient change and sustain talk holds up at the level of sequential response-by-response coding (e.g., Walthers et al., 2019).

Clinical Applications of MI

Chronic Illnesses

A primary use of MI in medical care has been to increase patients' health-relevant behaviors and decrease risk behaviors (Lundahl & Burke, 2009; Lundahl et al., 2010; Purath, Keck, & Fitzgerald, 2014). While this can be done in acute care—for example, to decrease risk of re-injury of patients treated in emergency departments (Havard, Shakeshaft, & Sanson-Fisher, 2008; Kohler

& Hofmann, 2015) and reduce rehospitalization (Poudel, Kavookjian, & Scalese, 2020)—the most common health applications have been in primary care (Barnes & Ivezaj, 2015; Morton et al., 2015; Olson, 2015; Purath et al., 2014; VanBuskirk & Wetherell, 2014) and the management of chronic conditions. MI is also a frequent component in brief interventions, such as Screening, Brief Intervention, and Referral to Treatment (SBIRT; Academic ED SBIRT Research Collaborative, 2007; Brooks et al., 2017).

Medication/Treatment Adherence

MI is often applied in managing chronic conditions (Schaefer & Kavookjian, 2017; VanBuskirk & Wetherell, 2014; Wagoner & Kavookjian, 2017), where a common obstacle is poor adherence with medication and self-care behaviors. MI has been used alone and in combination with cognitive-behavioral strategies to improve medication adherence (Easthall, Song, & Bhattacharya, 2013; Palacio et al., 2016; Spoelstra, Schueller, Hilton, & Ridenour, 2015; Teeter & Kavookjian, 2014; Zomahoun et al., 2016). Reviews have indicated that MI can be useful to improve screening or treatment adherence and in managing chronic conditions including:

- Asthma (Gayes & Steele, 2014; Gesinde & Harry, 2018)
- Cancer (Chan & So, 2021; Pourebrahim-Almadari et al., 2021; Pudkasam et al., 2021; Spencer & Wheeler, 2016)
- Cardiac rehabilitation (Bohplian & Bronas, 2022)
- Chronic pain (Alperstein & Sharpe, 2016)
- Diabetes (Dehghan-Nayeri, Ghaffari, Sadeghi, & Mozafarri, 2019)
- Heart disease (Cheng et al., 2015; Chew, Cheng, & Chair, 2019; Ghizzardi, Arrigoni, Dellafiore, Vellone, & Caruso, 2021; Lee, Choi, Yum, Yu, & Chair, 2016; Poudel et al., 2020; Sokalski, Hayden, Raffin Bouchal, Singh, & King-Shier, 2020; Thompson et al., 2011)
- HIV (Dillard, Zuniga, & Holstad, 2017; Hill & Kavookjian, 2012; Naar-King, Parsons, & Johnson, 2012)
- Hypertension (Conn, Ruppar, Chase, Enriquez, & Cooper, 2015; Cummings, Cooper, & Cassie, 2008; Lundahl et al., 2013; Ren, Yang, Browning, Thomas, & Liu, 2014; Rubak et al., 2005; VanBuskirk & Wetherell, 2014)
- Irritable bowel syndrome (Hill & Kavookjian, 2012)
- Multiple sclerosis (Dorstyn, Mathias, Bombardier, & Osborn, 2020)
- Obesity (Burgess, Hassmen, Welvaert, & Pumpa, 2017; Van Dorsten, 2007)

MI has also been used to promote health screening (S. J. Miller, Foran-Tuller, Ledergerber, & Jandorf, 2017) and water purification (Hettema et al., 2005; Lundahl et al., 2010), and has been linked to increased quality of life (Uzun & Özmaya, in press) and reduced mortality (Lundahl et al., 2013; Watkins et al., 2011). Rather than relying on MI alone, we recommend combining MI with other active treatment (Gesinde & Harry, 2018). There appears to be a synergistic effect when MI is combined with other evidence-based interventions, such that both can have larger and more enduring effects (Hettema et al., 2005).

Diabetes

Applications of MI in diabetes management are complex because there are so many target behaviors that can potentially benefit glycemic control (Steinberg & Miller, 2015). Reviews generally indicate that MI can impact diabetes-relevant self-care behaviors (Chapman et al., 2015; Cummings et al., 2008; Dehghan-Nayeri et al., 2019; Ekong & Kavookjian, 2016; Gayes & Steele, 2014; Martins & McNeil, 2009; Phillips & Guarnaccia, 2020; Song, Xu, & Sun, 2014; Thepwongsa, Muthukumar, & Kessomboon, 2017). Other reviews have questioned whether this is enough to lower HbA1c to a clinically significant extent (Concert, Burke, Eusebio, Slavin, & Shortridge-Baggett, 2012; Jones et al., 2014; Rubak et al., 2005; Winkley, Ismail, Landau, & Eisler, 2006), though more recent meta-analyses have found significant improvement in HbA1C for MI relative to controls (Berhe, Gebru, & Kahsay, 2020; Lestari, Wihastuti, & Ismail, 2021; McDaniel et al., 2021). In this regard, it is relevant to consider reviews of the effects of MI on specific behavioral components in managing diabetes and other chronic illnesses.

Weight Loss

Reviews of health behavior change research have supported a contribution of MI in reducing weight and body mass of children and adults (Amiri et al., 2021; Armstrong et al., 2011; Barnes & Ivezaj, 2015; DiRosa, 2010; Ekong & Kavookjian, 2016; Espinoza, San Carlos, Rojas, & Rioseco, 2019; Kao, Ling, Hawn, & Vu, 2021) and cholesterol (Cummings et al., 2008; Lundahl et al., 2013; Rubak et al., 2005); promoting dietary change (Borrelli, Tooley, & Scott-Sheldon, 2015; Stallings & Schneider, 2018; VanBuskirk & Wetherell, 2014; Van Dorsten, 2007) and readiness for change in eating disorders (Macdonald, Hibbs, Corfield, & Treasure, 2012). As with MI research more broadly, there is considerable variability in the effects of MI in treating obesity (Resnicow, Sonneville, & Naar, 2018). Evidence does not support the use of MI *alone* in promoting weight loss, but in combination with other effective interventions (Barrett, Begg, O'Halloran, & Kingsley, 2018; Vallabhan, Jimenez, & Kong, 2018).

Physical Activity

Reviews have reported a contribution of MI in increasing physical activity (Binder et al., 2019; Borrelli et al., 2015; DiRosa, 2010; Frost et al., 2016; Morton et al., 2015; Nuss, Moore, Nelson, & Li, 2021) including in people with chronic illnesses (O'Halloran et al., 2014; Sokalski et al., 2020) and in older adults (Cummings et al., 2008). A review in physiotherapy applications (McGrane, Galvin, Cusack, & Stokes, 2015) concluded that the addition of "motivational interventions can help adherence to exercise, have a positive effect on long-term exercise behavior, improve self-efficacy and reduce levels of activity limitation" (p. 1). Another review by Hollis and colleagues (2013) found no difference between MI and attention control. Again, we recommend combining MI with other evidence-based intervention components rather than relying on MI alone (Barrett et al., 2018; Burgess et al., 2017).

Parent–Child and Adolescent Health

In obstetric/gynecologic care, MI has shown promise in prenatal nutritional counseling (Castro, 2016), prevention of alcohol-exposed pregnancies (Handmaker & Wilbourne, 2001), and contraceptive use (Wilson et al., 2015). In pediatric care, reviews support MI in strengthening parent–child health behaviors (Borrelli et al., 2015; Erickson, Gerstle, & Feldstein, 2005; Gayes & Steele, 2014). In practicing MI directly with minors, evidence is strongest with adolescents and young adults (Cushing, Jensen, Miller, & Leffingwell, 2014; Naar-King & Suarez, 2011). MI has also been found useful in improving academic performance, school behavior, and educational motivation (Snape & Atkinson, 2016). With younger children, MI with parents is advised (Erickson et al., 2005), and reviews support the use of MI in strengthening parenting practices (Borrelli et al., 2015; Lundahl et al., 2010; Shah et al., 2018).

Substance Use Disorders

There is increasing evidence that substance use disorders can be treated and managed in medical care settings (Bertholet, Daeppen, Wietlisbach, Fleming, & Burnand, 2005; Bertholet et al., 2020; Saitz, Larson, La Belle, Richardson, & Samet, 2008). Treatment for alcohol/drug problems is gradually being integrated into mainstream health care, rather than relying exclusively on referral to specialist addiction programs (Miller & Weisner, 2002).

Alcohol

MI was originally developed to help patients stop or decrease risky and harmful alcohol use (Miller, 1983), and this is by far where the largest number of clinical trials and reviews have been published. Systematic reviews and meta-analyses include: Appiah-Brempong, Okyere, Owusu-Addo, & Cross, 2014; Barnett, Sussman, Smith, Rohrbach, & Spruijt-Metz, 2012; Bertholet et al., 2005; Bien, Miller, & Tonigan, 1993; Branscum & Sharma, 2010; Burke, Arkowitz, & Menchola, 2003; Burke, Dunn, Atkins, & Phelps, 2004; DiClemente et al., 2017; Frost et al., 2016; J. Hettema et al., 2005; Jensen et al., 2011; Jiang, Wu, & Gao, 2017; Kohler & Hofmann, 2015; Lenz, Rosenbaum, & Sheperis, 2016; Lundahl & Burke, 2009; Lundahl et al., 2010, 2013; McKenzie et al., 2015; McQueen, Howe, Allan, Mains, & Hardy, 2011; Merz, Baptista, & Haller, 2015; Miller & Wilbourne, 2002; Miller, Wilbourne, & Hettema, 2003; Morton et al., 2015; Moyer, Finney, Swearingen, & Vergun, 2002; Rubak et al., 2005; Samson & Tanner-Smith, 2015; Steinka-Fry, Tanner-Smith, & Hennessy, 2015; Tanner-Smith & Lipsey, 2015; Tanner-Smith & Risser, 2016; Vasilaki, Hosier, & Cox, 2006; and Wilk, Jensen, & Havighurst, 1997. The impact of MI on heavy drinking is well documented across a wide variety of populations and settings. Two meta-analyses claimed less efficacy of MI with youth (Foxcroft et al., 2016) and college students (Huh et al., 2015), though others have specifically supported the efficacy of MI with these populations (Appiah-Brempong et al., 2014; Barnett et al., 2012; Branscum & Sharma, 2010; Jensen et al., 2011; Kohler & Hofmann, 2015; Mun, Atkins, & Walters, 2015; Samson & Tanner-Smith, 2015; Steinka-Fry et al., 2015; Tanner-Smith & Lipsey, 2015; Tanner-Smith & Risser, 2016).

Tobacco

All four reviews prior to 2006 concluded little or no efficacy of MI to impact smoking cessation (Burke et al., 2003, 2004; Hettema et al., 2005; Rubak et al., 2005). In marked contrast, most reviews since 2008 found support for MI as an evidence-based intervention for smokers (Cummings et al., 2008; DiClemente et al., 2017; Frost et al., 2016; Gesinde & Harry, 2018; Heckman, Egleston, & Hofmann, 2010; Hettema & Hendricks, 2010; Lai, Cahill, Qin, & Tang, 2010; Lee et al., 2016; Lundahl & Burke, 2009; Lundahl et al., 2010, 2013; McKenzie et al., 2015; Poudel & Kavookjian, 2018). One meta-analysis (Lindson, Thompson, Ferrey, Lambert, & Aveyard, 2019; Lindson-Hawley, Thompson, & Begh, 2015) concluded uncertainty about MI's effect on smoking cessation.

Marijuana

Reviews and meta-analyses to date have consistently supported the efficacy of MI in addressing cannabis use disorders (DiClemente et al., 2017; Gates, Sabioni, Copeland, Le Foll, & Gowing, 2016; Grenard, Ames, Pentz, & Sussman, 2006; Halladay et al., 2019; Lundahl & Burke, 2009; Lundahl et al., 2010, 2013). It is worth noting, however, that with rapid transitions in the availability, legality, variety, and potency of cannabis products in the United States, findings may change.

Illicit Drugs

When reviews evaluate the efficacy of MI for substance use disorders in general, they usually support efficacy. This can be misleading, however, because the vast majority of these clinical trials are with alcohol, tobacco, or marijuana. The efficacy of MI is currently less clear with methamphetamine, opioids (DiClemente et al., 2017), benzodiazepines (Darker, Sweeney, Barry, Farrell, & Donnelly-Swift, 2015), and illicit drugs more generally (Jiang et al., 2017; Li, Zhu, Tse, Tse, & Wong, 2016).

Preventive Dentistry

Beyond the relevance of oral hygiene in preventing tooth loss, chronic periodontitis is persuasively linked to cardiovascular disease independent from other risk factors (Dietrich et al., 2017; Fisher, Borgnakke, & Taylor, 2010). Gum disease is preventable with tooth brushing and flossing, yet poor adherence is common. Reviews of clinical trials generally support the efficacy of MI in promoting oral hygiene and preventing gum disease, though as with other clinical applications, evidence is inconsistent (Albino & Tiwari, 2016; Borrelli et al., 2015; Cascaes, Bielemann, Clark, & Barros, 2014; Gao, Lo, Kot, & Chan, 2014; Kay, Vascott, Hocking, & Nield, 2016; Kopp, Ramseier, Ratka-Krüger, & Woelber, 2017; Lundahl et al., 2013; Martins & McNeil, 2009). MI may also be useful in parental education to prevent early childhood caries (Colvara et al., 2021; Faghihian, Faghihian, Kazemi, Tarrahi, & Zakizade, 2020).

Mental Health

Applications of MI are also growing in the treatment of psychological problems (Arkowitz, Miller, & Rollnick, 2015). Beyond the large literature on substance use disorders discussed above, reviews have appeared supporting a role for MI in treating anxiety disorders (Marker & Norton, 2018; Randall & McNeil, 2017) and depression (Cheng et al., 2015; Riper et al., 2014), and in managing severe mental disorders (Drymalski & Campbell, 2009; Wong-Anuchit, Chantamit-o-pas, Schneider, & Mills, 2019).

Summary

The number of clinical issues to which MI has been applied is impressive. With small to medium effect sizes on average, there is large variability in findings, from no effect to large effects. Studies of MI often have provided insufficient description or documentation of the intervention to judge whether MI was actually practiced with fidelity (Mack, Wilson, Bell, & Kelley, 2020; Miller & Rollnick, 2014). Outcomes vary across studies, sites, and providers within sites. Interpretation is difficult without documentation of what was actually delivered, and we know that providers' belief that they are practicing MI bears little relationship to observer ratings. It is clear that MI *can* influence health behavior change across a wide range of clinical problems, and that part of the variability in outcomes is related to fidelity of practice. Randomized clinical trials offer one piece of the puzzle, but it is likely that advances in the understanding of MI will require other research designs linking observed processes with treatment outcomes.

References

Academic ED SBIRT Research Collaborative. (2007). The impact of Screening, Brief Intervention, and Referral for Treatment on Emergency Department patients' alcohol use. *Annals of Emergency Medicine, 50*(6), 699–710, 710.e1–e6.

Albino, J., & Tiwari, T. (2016). Preventing childhood caries: A review of recent behavioral research. *Journal of Dental Research, 95*(1), 35–42.

Alperstein, D., & Sharpe, L. (2016). The efficacy of motivational interviewing in adults with chronic pain: A meta-analysis and systematic review. *Journal of Pain, 17*(4), 393–403.

Amiri, P., Mansouri-Tehrani, M. M., Khalili-Chelik, A., Karimi, M., Jalali-Farahani, S., Amouzegar, A., & Kazemian, E. (2021). Does motivational interviewing improve the weight management process in adolescents?: A systematic review and meta-analysis. *International Journal of Behavioral Medicine, 29*(1), 78-103.

Apodaca, T. R., Jackson, K. M., Borsari, B., Magill, M., Longabaugh, R., Mastroleo, N. R., & Barnett, N. P. (2016). Which individual therapist behaviors elicit client change talk and sustain talk in motivational interviewing? *Journal of Substance Abuse Treatment, 61,* 60–65.

Apodaca, T. R., & Longabaugh, R. (2009). Mechanisms of change in motivational interviewing: A review and preliminary evaluation of the evidence. *Addiction, 104*(5), 705–715.

Appiah-Brempong, E., Okyere, P., Owusu-Addo, E., & Cross, R. (2014). Motivational interviewing interventions and alcohol abuse among college students: A systematic review. *American Journal of Health Promotion, 29*(1), e32–e42.

Arkowitz, H., Miller, W. R., & Rollnick, S. (Eds.). (2015). *Motivational interviewing in the treatment of psychological probems* (2nd ed.). Guilford Press.

Armstrong, M. J., Mottershead, R. A., Ronksley, P. E., Sigal, R. J., Campbell, T. S., & Hemmelgarn, B. R. (2011). Motivational interviewing to improve weight loss in overweight and/or obese patients: A systematic review and meta-analysis of randomized clinical trials. *Obesity Reviews, 12*(9), 709–723.

Aveyard, P., Begh, R., Parsons, A., & West, R. (2012). Brief opportunistic smoking cessation interventions: A systematic review and meta-analysis to compare advice to quit and offer of assistance. *Addiction, 107*(6), 1066–1073.

Bahafzallah, L., Hayden, K. A., Bouchal, S. R., Singh, P., & King-Shier, K. M. (2020). Motivational interviewing in ethnic populations. *Journal of Immigrant and Minority Health, 22*(4), 816–851.

Barnes, R. D., & Ivezaj, V. (2015). A systematic review of motivational interviewing for weight loss among adults in primary care. *Obesity Reviews, 16*(4), 304–318.

Barnett, E., Sussman, S., Smith, C., Rohrbach, L. A., & Spruijt-Metz, D. (2012). Motivational Interviewing for adolescent substance use: A review of the literature. *Addictive Behaviors, 37*(12), 1325–1334.

Barrett, S., Begg, S., O'Halloran, P., & Kingsley, M. (2018). Integrated motivational interviewing and cognitive behaviour therapy for lifestyle mediators of overweight and obesity in community-dwelling adults: A systematic review and meta-analyses. *BMC Public Health 18*(1160).

Barry, M. J., & Edgman-Levitan, S. (2012). Shared decision making—Pinnacle of patient-centered care. *New England Journal of Medicine, 366*(9), 780–781.

Barwick, M. A., Bennett, L. M., Johnson, S. N., McGowan, J., & Moore, J. E. (2012). Training health and mental health professionals in motivational interviewing: A systematic review. *Children and Youth Services Review, 34*(9), 1786–1795.

Berhe, K. K., Gebru, H. B., & Kahsay, H. B. (2020). Effect of motivational interviewing intervention on HgbA1C and depression in people with type 2 diabetes mellitus (systematic review and meta-analysis). *PloS One, 15*(10), e0240839.

Bertholet, N., Daeppen, J. B., Wietlisbach, V., Fleming, M., & Burnand, B. (2005). Reduction of alcohol consumption by brief alcohol intervention in primary care: Systematic review and meta-analysis. *Archives of Internal Medicine, 165*(9), 986–995.

Bertholet, N., Meli, S., Palfai, T. P., Cheng, D. M., Alford, D. P., Bernstein, J., . . . Saitz, R. (2020). Screening and brief intervention for lower-risk drug use in primary care: A pilot randomized trial. *Drug and Alcohol Dependence, 213*(108001).

Bien, T. H., Miller, W. R., & Tonigan, J. S. (1993). Brief interventions for alcohol problems: A review. *Addiction, 88*, 315–336.

Binder, J., Hannum, C., McCarthy, C., McLeod, E., Overpeck, J., Kaiser, L., & Potvin, M.-C. (2019). *A systematic review of the efficacy of motivational interviewing on occupational performance.* Student Papers & Posters. https://jdc.jefferson.edu/student_papers/32.

Bischof, G., Bischof, A., & Rumpf, H.-J. (2021). Motivational interviewing: An evidence-based approach for use in medical practice. *Deutsches Ärzteblatt International, 118*(7), 109–115.

Boccio, M., Sanna, R. S., Adams, S. R., Goler, N. C., Brown, S. D., Neugebauer, S., . . . Schmittdiel, J. A. (2017). Telephone-based coaching: A comparison of tobacco cessation programs in an integrated health care system. *American Journal of Health Promotion, 31*(2), 136–142.

Bohplian, S., & Bronas, U. G. (2022). Motivational strategies and concepts to increase participation and adherence in cardiac rehabilitation: An integrative review. *Journal of Cardiopulmonary Rehabilitation and Prevention 42*(2), 75-83.

Borrelli, B., Tooley, E. M., & Scott-Sheldon, L. A. (2015). Motivational interviewing for parent–child health interventions: A systematic review and meta-analysis. *Pediatric Dentistry, 37*(3), 254–265.

Branscum, P., & Sharma, M. (2010). A systematic review of motivational interviewing-based interventions targeting problematic drinking among college students. *Alcoholism Treatment Quarterly, 28*(1), 63–77.

Brooks, A. C., Carpenedo, C. M., Lauby, J., Metzger, D., Byrne, E., Favor, K., & Kirby, K. C. (2017). Expanded brief intervention for substance use in primary care. *Drug and Alcohol Dependence, 171*, e26–e27.

Burgess, E., Hassmen, P., Welvaert, M., & Pumpa, K. L. (2017). Behavioural treatment strategies improve adherence to lifestyle intervention programmes in adults with obesity: A systematic review and meta-analysis. *Clinical Obesity, 7*(2), 105–114.

Burke, B. L., Arkowitz, H., & Menchola, M. (2003). The efficacy of motivational interviewing: A meta-analysis of controlled clinical trials. *Journal of Consulting and Clinical Psychology, 71*(5), 843–861.

Burke, B. L., Dunn, C. W., Atkins, D. C., & Phelps, J. S. (2004). The emerging evidence base for motivational interviewing: A meta-analytic and qualitative inquiry. *Journal of Cognitive Psychotherapy: An International Quarterly, 18*(4), 309–322.

Cascaes, A. M., Bielemann, R. M., Clark, V. L., & Barros, A. J. D. (2014). Effectiveness of motivational interviewing at improving oral health: A systematic review. *Revista de Saúde Pública, 48*(1), 142–153.

Castro, K. M. G. (2016). *Impact of prenatal motivational interviewing on health status and health behavior related with nutrition: A systematic review.* Master's thesis, Kent State University, Kent, OH.

Chan, D. N. S., & So, W. K. W. (2021). Effectiveness of motivational interviewing in enhancing cancer screening uptake amongst average-risk individuals: A systematic review. *International Journal of Nursing Studies, 113*, 103786.

Channon, S. J., Huws-Thomas, M. V., Rollnick, S., Hood, K., Cannings-John, R. L., Rogers, C. R., & Gregory, J. W. (2007). A multicenter randomized controlled trial of motivational interviewing in teenagers with diabetes. *Diabetes Care, 30*(6), 1390–1395.

Chapman, A., Liu, S., Merkouris, S., Enticott, J. C., Yang, H., Browning, C. J., & Thomas, S. A. (2015). Psychological interventions for the management of glycemic and psychological outcomes of type 2 diabetes mellitus in China: A systematic review and meta-analyses of randomized controlled trials. *Frontiers in Public Health, 3*, 252.

Cheng, D., Qu, Z., Huang, J., Xiao, Y., Luo, H., & Wang, J. (2015). Motivational interviewing for improving recovery after stroke. *Cochrane Database of Systematic Reviews*, Issue 6, Article No. CD011398.

Chew, H. S. J., Cheng, H. Y., & Chair, S. Y. (2019). The suitability of motivational interviewing versus cognitive behavioural interventions on improving self-care in patients with heart failure: A literature review and discussion paper. *Applied Nursing Research, 45*, 17–22.

Colvara, B. C., Faustino-Silva, D. D., Meyer, E., Hugo, F. N., Celeste, R. K., & Hilgert, J. B. (2021). Motivational interviewing for preventing early childhood caries: A systematic review and meta-analysis. *Community Dentistry and Oral Epidemiology, 49*(1), 10–16.

Concert, C. M., Burke, R. E., Eusebio, A. M., Slavin, E. A., & Shortridge-Baggett, L. M. (2012). The effectiveness of motivational interviewing on glycemic control for adults with type 2 diabetes mellitus (DM2): A systematic review. *JBI Library of Systematic Reviews, 10*(42, Suppl.), 1–17.

Conn, V. S., Ruppar, T. M., Chase, J. A., Enriquez, M., & Cooper, P. S. (2015). Interventions to improve medication adherence in hypertensive patients: Systematic review and meta-analysis. *Current Hypertension Reports, 17*(12), 94.

Copeland, L., McNamara, R., Kelson, M., & Simpson, S. (2015). Mechanisms of change within motivational interviewing in relation to health behaviors outcomes: A systematic review. *Patient Education and Counseling, 98*(4), 401–411.

Cummings, S. M., Cooper, R. L., & Cassie, K. M. (2008). Motivational interviewing to affect behavioral change in older adults. *Research on Social Work Practice, 19*(2), 195–204.

Cushing, C. C., Jensen, C. D., Miller, M. B., & Leffingwell, T. R. (2014). Meta-analysis of motivational interviewing for adolescent health behavior: Efficacy beyond substance use. *Journal of Consulting and Clinical Psychology, 82*(6), 1212–1218.

Darker, C. D., Sweeney, B. P., Barry, J. M., Farrell, M. F., & Donnelly-Swift, E. (2015). Psychosocial interventions for benzodiazepine harmful use, abuse or dependence. *Cochrane Dataabse of Systematic Reviews*, Issue 5, Article No. CD009652.

de Almeida Neto, A. C. (2017). Understanding motivational interviewing: An evolutionary perspective. *Evolutionary Psychological Science, 3*(4), 379–389

Deci, E. L., & Ryan, R. M. (2000). The "what" and "why" of goal pursuits: Human needs and the self-determination of behavior. *Psychological Inquiry, 11*, 227–268.

Dehghan-Nayeri, N., Ghaffari, F., Sadeghi, T., & Mozaffari, N. (2019). Effects of motivational interviewing on adherence to treatment regimens among patients with type 1 diabetes: A systematic review. *Diabetes Spectrum, 32*(2), 112–117.

de Roten, Y., Zimmerman, G., Ortega, D., & Despland, J. N. (2013).

Meta-analysis of the effects of MI training on clinicians' behavior. *Journal of Substance Abuse Treatment, 45*(2), 155–162.

DiClemente, C. C., Corno, C. M., Graydon, M. M., Wiprovnick, A. E., & Knoblach, D. J. (2017). Motivational interviewing, enhancement, and brief interventions over the last decade: A review of reviews of efficacy and effectiveness. *Psychology of Addictive Behaviors, 31*(8), 862–887.

Dietrich, T., Webb, I., Stenhouse, L., Pattni, A., Ready, D., Wanyonyi, K. L., . . . Gallagher, J. E. (2017). Evidence summary: The relationship between oral and cardiovascular disease. *British Dental Journal, 222*, 381–385.

Dillard, J. P., & Shen, L. (2005). On the nature of reactance and its role in persuasive health communication. *Communication Monographs, 72*(2), 144–168.

Dillard, P. K., Zuniga, J. A., & Holstad, M. M. (2017). An integrative review of the efficacy of motivational interviewing in HIV management. *Patient Education and Counseling, 100*(4), 636–646.

DiRosa, L. C. (2010). *Motivational interviewing to treat overweight/obesity: A meta-analysis of relevant research.* Unpublished doctoral dissertation, Wilmington University, New Castle, DE.

Doran, G. T. (1981). There's a S.M.A.R.T. way to write management's goals and objectives. *Management Review, 70*, 35–36.

Dorstyn, D. S., Mathias, J. L., Bombardier, C. H., & Osborn, A. J. (2020). Motivational interviewing to promote health outcomes and behaviour change in multiple sclerosis: A systematic review. *Clinical Rehabilitation, 34*(3), 299–309.

Drymalski, W. M., & Campbell, T. C. (2009). A review of motivational interviewing to enhance adherence to antipsychotic medication in patients with schizophrenia: Evidence and recommendations. *Journal of Mental Health, 18*, 6–15.

Dunhill, D., Schmidt, S., & Klein, R. (2014). Motivational interviewing interventions in graduate medical education: A systematic review of the evidence. *Journal of Graduate Medical Education, 6*(2), 222–236.

Easthall, C., Song, F., & Bhattacharya, D. (2013). A meta-analysis of cognitive-based behaviour change techniques as interventions to improve medication adherence. *BMJ Open, 3*(8), e002749.

Egan, G. (2013). *The skilled helper: A problem-management and opportunity-developing approach to helping* (10th ed.). Cengage Learning.

Ekong, G., & Kavookjian, J. (2016). Motivational interviewing and outcomes in adults with type 2 diabetes: A systematic review. *Patient Education and Counseling, 99*(6), 944–952.

Elliott, R., Bohart, A. C., Watson, J. C., & Murphy, D. (2018). Therapist empathy and client outcome: An updated meta-analysis. *Psychotherapy, 55*(4), 399–410.

Erickson, S. J., Gerstle, M., & Feldstein, S. W. (2005). Brief interventions and motivational interviewing with children, adolescents, and their parents in pediatric health care settings: A review. *Archives of Pediatrics & Adolescent Medicine, 159*(12), 1173–1180.

Espinoza, P. G., San Carlos, N. G., Rojas, D. N., & Rioseco, R. C. (2019). Is the individual motivational interviewing effective in overweight and obesity treatment?: A systematic review. *Atención Primaria 51*(9), 548–561.

Faghihian, R., Faghihian, E., Kazemi, A., Tarrahi, M. J., & Zakizade, M. (2020). Impact of motivational interviewing on early childhood caries: A systematic review and meta-analysis. *Journal of the American Dental Association, 151*(9), 650–659.

Fisher, M. A., Borgnakke, W. S., & Taylor, G. W. (2010). Periodontal disease as a risk marker in coronary heart disease and chronic kidney disease. *Current Opinion in Nephrology and Hypertension, 19*(6), 519–526.

Foxcroft, D. R., Coombes, L., Wood, S., Allen, D., Almeida Santimano, N. M. L., & Moreira, M. T. (2016). Motivational interviewing for the prevention of alcohol misuse in young adults. *Cochrane Database of Systematic Reviews*, Issue 7, Article No. CD007025.

Frost, H., Campbell, P., Maxwell, M., O'Carroll, R., Dombrowski, S., Cheyne, H., . . . Pollock, A. (2016). Effectiveness of motivational interviewing on adult behaviour change in health and social care settings: An overview of reviews. *Physiotherapy, 102*(Suppl. 1), e59–e60.

Frost, H., Campbell, P., Maxwell, M., O'Carroll, R. E., Dombrowski, S. U., Williams, B., . . . Pollock, A. (2018). Effectiveness of motivational interviewing on adult behaviour change in health and social care settings: A systematic review of reviews. *PloS One, 13*(10), e020489.

Gao, X., Lo, E. C. Y., Kot, S. C. C., & Chan, K. C. W. (2014). Motivational interviewing in improving oral health: A systematic review of randomized controlled trials. *Journal of Periodontology, 85*(3), 426–437.

Gates, P. J., Sabioni, P., Copeland, J., Le Foll, B., & Gowing, L. (2016). Psychosocial interventions for cannabis use disorder. *Cochrane Database of Systematic Reviews*, Issue 5, Article No. CD005336.

Gayes, L. A., & Steele, R. G. (2014). A meta-analysis of motivational interviewing interventions for pediatric health behavior change. *Journal of Consulting and Clinical Psychology, 82*(3), 521–535.

Gesinde, B., & Harry, S. (2018). The use of motivational interviewing in improving medication adherence for individuals with asthma: A systematic review. *Perspectives in Public Health, 138*(6), 329–335.

Ghizzardi, G., Arrigoni, C., Dellafiore, F., Vellone, E., & Caruso, R. (2021). Efficacy of motivational interviewing on enhancing self-care behaviors among patients with chronic heart failure: A systematic review and meta-analysis of randomized controlled trials. *Heart Failure Reviews*. Epub ahead of print.

Glynn, L. H., & Moyers, T. B. (2010). Chasing change talk: The clinician's role in evoking client language about change. *Journal of Substance Abuse Treatment, 39*(1), 65–70.

Gollwitzer, P. M. (1999). Implementation intentions: Simple effects of simple plans. *American Psychologist, 54*(7), 493–503.

Gordon, T., & Edwards, W. S. (1997). *Making the patient your partner: Communication skills for doctors and other caregivers*. Auburn House.

Grenard, J. L., Ames, S. L., Pentz, M. A., & Sussman, S. (2006). Motivational interviewing with adolescents and young adults for drug-related problems. *International Journal of Adolescent Medicine and Health, 18*(1), 53–67.

Hall, K., Staiger, P. K., Simpson, A., Best, D., & Lubman, D. I. (2016). After 30 years of dissemination, have we achieved sustained practice change in motivational interviewing? *Addiction, 111*(7), 1144–1150.

Halladay, J., Scherer, J., MacKillop, J., Woock, R., Petker, T., Linton, V., & Munn, C. (2019). Brief interventions for cannabis use in emerging adults: A systematic review, meta-analysis, and evidence map. *Drug and Alcohol Dependence, 204*(107565).

Handmaker, N. S., & Wilbourne, P. (2001). Motivational interventions in prenatal clinics. *Alcohol Research & Health, 25*(3), 219–229.

Hart, J. T. (1971). The inverse care law. *Lancet, 1*(7696), 405–412.

Havard, A., Shakeshaft, A., & Sanson-Fisher, R. (2008). Systematic review and meta-analyses of strategies targeting alcohol problems in emergency departments: Interventions reduce alcohol-related injuries. *Addiction, 103*(3), 368–376; discussion, 377–368.

Heckman, C. J., Egleston, B. L., & Hofmann, M. T. (2010). Efficacy of motivational interviewing for smoking cessation: A systematic review and meta-analysis. *Tobacco Control, 19*(5), 410–416.

Hettema, J., Steele, J., & Miller, W. R. (2005). Motivational interviewing. *Annual Review of Clinical Psychology, 1*, 91–111.

Hettema, J. E., & Hendricks, P. S. (2010). Motivational interviewing for smoking cessation: A meta-analytic review. *Journal of Consulting and Clinical Psychology, 78*(6), 868–884.

Hibbard, J. H., Mahoney, E. R., Stock, R., & Tusler, M. (2007). Do increases in patient activation result in improved self-management behaviors? *Health Services Research, 42*(4), 1443–1463.

Hill, S., & Kavookjian, J. (2012). Motivational interviewing as a behavioral intervention to increase HAART adherence in patients who are HIV-positive: A systematic review of the literature. *AIDS Care, 24*(5), 583–592.

Hollis, J. L., Williams, L. T., Collins, C. E., & Morgan, P. J. (2013). Effectiveness of interventions using motivational interviewing for dietary and physical activity modification in adults: A systematic review. *JBI Database of Systematic Reviews & Implementation Reports, 11*(5), 1–27.

Huh, D., Mun, E. Y., Larimer, M. E., White, H. R., Ray, A. E., Rhew, I. C., . . . Atkins, D. C. (2015). Brief motivational interventions for college student drinking may not be as powerful as we think: An individual participant-level data meta-analysis. *Alcoholism: Clinical and Experimental Research, 39*(5), 919–931.

Hurlocker, M. C., Madson, M. B., & Schumacher, J. A. (2020). Motivational interviewing quality assurance: A systematic review of assessment tools across research contexts. *Clinical Psychology Review, 82*, Article 101909.

Jensen, C. D., Cushing, C. C., Aylward, B. S., Craig, J. T., Sorell, D. M., & Steele, R. G. (2011). Effectiveness of motivational interviewing interventions for adolescent substance use behavior change: A meta-analytic review. *Journal of Consulting and Clinical Psychology, 79*(4), 433–440.

Jiang, S., Wu, L., & Gao, X. (2017). Beyond face-to-face individual counseling: A systematic review on alternative modes of motivational interviewing in substance abuse treatment and prevention. *Addictive Behaviors, 73*, 216–235.

Jones, A., Gladstone, B. P., Lübeck, M., Lindekilde, N., Upton, D., & Vach, W. (2014). Motivational interventions in the management of HbA1c levels: A systematic review and meta-analysis. *Primary Care Diabetes, 8*(2), 91–100.

Kaczmarek, T., Kavanagh, D., Lazzarini, P. A., Warnock, J., & Van Netten, J. J. (2021). Training diabetes healthcare practitioners in motivational interviewing: A systematic review. *Health Psychology Review.* Epub ahead of print.

Kaltman, S., & Tankersley, A. (2020). Teaching motivational interviewing to medical students: A systematic review. *Academic Medicine, 95*(3), 458–469.

Kao, T. A., Ling, J., Hawn, R., & Vu, C. (2021). The effects of motivational interviewing on children's body mass index and fat distributions: A systematic review and meta-analysis. *Obesity Reviews, 22*(10), e13308.

Kay, E. J., Vascott, D., Hocking, A., & Nield, H. (2016). Motivational interviewing in general dental practice: A review of the evidence. *British Dental Journal, 221*(12), 785–791.

Keeley, R., Engel, M., Reed, A., Brody, D., & Burke, B. L. (2018). Toward an emerging role for motivational interviewing in primary care. *Psychiatry in Primary Care, 20*(41).

Kohler, S., & Hofmann, A. (2015). Can motivational interviewing in emergency care reduce alcohol consumption in young people?: A systematic review and meta-analysis. *Alcohol and Alcoholism, 50*(2), 107–117.

Kopp, S. L., Ramseier, C. A., Ratka-Krüger, P., & Woelber, J. P. (2017). Motivational interviewing as an adjunct to periodontal therapy—A systematic review. *Frontiers in Psychology, 8*(279).

Kraus, M. W. (2017). Voice-only communication enhances empathic accuracy. *American Psychologist, 72*(7), 644–654.

Lai, D. T., Cahill, K., Qin, Y., & Tang, J. L. (2010). Motivational interviewing for smoking cessation. *Cochrane Database of Systematic Reviews*, Issue 1, Article No. CD006936.

Lane, C., Butterworth, S., & Speck, L. (2013). Motivational interviewing for people with chronic health conditions. In C. C. Wagner & K. Ingersoll (Eds.), *Motivational interviewing in groups* (pp. 314–331). Guilford Press.

Lee, C. S., Baird, J., Longabaugh, R., Nirenberg, T. D., Mello, M. J., & Woolard, R. (2010). Change plan as an active ingredient of brief motivational interventions for reducing negative consequences of drinking in hazardous drinking emergency-department patients. *Journal of Studies on Alcohol and Drugs, 71*, 726–733.

Lee, C. S., Colby, S. M., Rohsenow, D. J., Martin, R., Rosales, R., McCallum, T. T., . . . Cortés, D. E. (2019). A randomized controlled trial of motivational interviewing tailored for heavy drinking latinxs. *Journal of Consulting and Clinical Psychology, 87*(9), 815–830.

Lee, W. W. M., Choi, K. C., Yum, R., Yu, D. S. F., & Chair, S. Y. (2016). Effectiveness of motivational interviewing on lifestyle modification and health outcomes of clients at risk or diagnosed with cardiovascular diseases: A systematic review. *International Journal of Nursing Studies, 53*(1), 331–341.

Lenz, A. S., Rosenbaum, L., & Sheperis, D. (2016). Meta-analysis of randomized controlled trials of motivational enhancement therapy for reducing substance use. *Journal of Addictions & Offender Counseling, 37*(2), 66–86.

Lestari, S. P., Wihastuti, T. A., & Ismail, D. D. S. L. (2021). The effectiveness of motivational interviewing on the self management of type 2 diabetes mellitus patients: A systematic review. *Jurnal Kedokteran Brawijaya, 31*(4).

Li, L., Zhu, S., Tse, N., Tse, S., & Wong, P. (2016). Effectiveness of motivational interiewing to reduce illicit drug use in adolescents: A systematic review and meta-analysis. *Addiction, 111*(5), 795–805.

Lindson, N., Thompson,T. P., Ferrey, A., Lambert, J. D., & Aveyard, P. (2019). Motivational interviewing for smoking cessation. *Cochrane Database of Systematic Reviews*, Issue 7, Article No. CD006936.

Lindson-Hawley, N., Thompson, T. P., & Begh, R. (2015). Motivational interviewing for smoking cessation. *Cochrane Database of Systematic Reviews*, Issue 3, Article No. CD006936.

Logel, C., & Cohen, G. L. (2012). The role of the self in physical health: Testing the effect of a values-affirmation intervention on weight loss. *Psychological Science, 23*(1), 53–55.

Lundahl, B., & Burke, B. L. (2009). The effectiveness and applicability of motivational interviewing: A practice-friendly review of four meta-analyses. *Journal of Clinical Psychology, 65*(11), 1232–1245.

Lundahl, B., Moleni, T., Burke, B. L., Butters, R., Tollefson, D., Butler, C., & Rollnick, S. (2013). Motivational interviewing in medical care settings: A systematic review and meta-analysis of randomized controlled trials. *Patient Education and Counseling, 93*(2), 157–168.

Lundahl, B. W., Kunz, C., Brownell, C., Tollefson, D., & Burke, B. L. (2010). A meta-analysis of motivational interviewing: Twenty-five years of empirical studies. *Research on Social Work Practice, 20*(2), 137–160.

Macdonald, P., Hibbs, R., Corfield, F., & Treasure, J. (2012). The use of motivational interviewing in eating disorders: A systematic review. *Psychiatry Research, 200*(1), 1–11.

Mack, D. E., Wilson, P. M., Bell, C., & Kelley, C. (2020). The devil is always in the details: Intervention description as applied to motivational interviewing and physical activity. *Canadian Journal of Behavioural Science, 52*(1), 29–35.

Magill, M., Apodaca, T. R., Borsari, B., Gaume, J., Hoadley, A., Gordon, R. E. F., . . . Moyers, T. (2018). A meta-analysis of motivational interviewing process: Technical, relational, and conditional process models of change. *Journal of Consulting and Clinical Psychology, 86*(2), 140–157.

Magill, M., Bernstein, M. H., Hoadley, A., Borsari, B., Apodaca, T. R., Gaume, J., & Tonigan, J. S. (2019). Do what you say and say what you are going to do: A preliminary meta-analysis of client change and sustain talk subtypes in motivational interviewing. *Psychotherapy Research, 29*(7), 860–869.

Magill, M., Gaume, J., Apodaca, T. R., Walthers, J., Mastroleo, N. R., Borsari, B., & Longabaugh, R. (2014). The technical hypothesis of motivational interviewing: A meta-analysis of MI's key causal model. *Journal of Consulting and Clinical Psychology, 82*(6), 973–983.

Marker, I., & Norton, P. J. (2018). The efficacy of incorporating motivational interviewing to cognitive behavior therapy for anxiety disorders: A review and meta-analysis. *Clinical Psychology Review, 62*, 1–10.

Marshall, C., & Nielsen, A. S. (2020). *Motivational interviewing for leaders in the helping professions: Facilitating change in organizations.* Guilford Press.

Martino, S., & Santa Ana, E. J. (2013). Motivational interviewing groups for dually diagnosed patients. In C. C. Wagner & K. Ingersoll (Eds.), *Motivational interviewing in groups* (pp. 297–313). Guilford Press.

Martins, R. K., & McNeil, D. W. (2009). Review of motivational interviewing in promoting health behaviors. *Clinical Psychology Review, 29*(4), 283–293.

McDaniel, C. C., Kavookjian, J., & Whitley, H. P. (2021). Telehealth delivery of motivational interviewing for diabetes management: A systematic review of randomized controlled trials. *Patient Education and Counseling.* Epub ahead of print.

McGrane, N., Galvin, R., Cusack, T., & Stokes, E. (2015). Addition of motivational interventions to exercise and traditional physiotherapy: A review and meta-analysis. *Physiotherapy, 101*(1), 1–12.

McKenzie, K. J., Pierce, D., & Gunn, J. M. (2015). A systematic review of motivational interviewing in healthcare: The potential of motivational interviewing to address the lifestyle factors relevant to multimorbidity. *Journal of Comorbidity, 5*(1), 162–174.

McQueen, J., Howe, T. E., Allan, L., Mains, D., & Hardy, V. (2011). Brief interventions for heavy alcohol users admitted to general hospital wards. *Cochrane Database of Systematic Reviews*, Issue 8, Article No. CD005191.

Merz, V., Baptista, J., & Haller, D. M. (2015). Brief interventions to prevent recurrence and alcohol-related problems in young adults admitted to the emergency ward following an alcohol-related event: A systematic review. *Journal of Epidemiology & Community Health, 69*(9), 912–917.

Miller, S. J., Foran-Tuller, K., Ledergerber, J., & Jandorf, L. (2017). Motivational interviewing to improve health screening uptake: A systematic review. *Patient Education and Counseling, 100*(2), 190–198.

Miller, W. R. (2018). *Listening well: The art of empathic understanding.* Wipf & Stock.

Miller, W. R., & Mount, K. A. (2001). A small study of training in motivational interviewing: Does one workshop change clinician and client behavior? *Behavioural and Cognitive Psychotherapy, 29*, 457–471.

Miller, W. R., & Moyers, T. B. (2021). *Effective psychotherapists: Clinical skills that improve client outcomes.* Guilford Press.

Miller, W. R., & Rollnick, S. (2013). *Motivational interviewing: Helping people change* (3rd ed.). Guilford Press.

Miller, W. R., & Rollnick, S. (2014). The effectiveness and ineffectiveness of complex behavioral interventions: Impact of treatment fidelity. *Contemporary Clinical Trials, 37*(2), 234–241.

Miller, W. R., & Rose, G. S. (2015). Motivational interviewing and decisional balance: Contrasting responses to client ambivalence. *Behavioural and Cognitive Psychotherapy, 43*(2), 129–141.

Miller, W. R., & Weisner, C. (Eds.). (2002). *Changing substance abuse through health and social systems.* Kluwer/Plenum.

Miller, W. R., & Wilbourne, P. L. (2002). Mesa Grande: A methodological analysis of clinical trials of treatment for alcohol use disorders. *Addiction, 97*(3), 265–277.

Miller, W. R., Wilbourne, P. L., & Hettema, J. (2003). What works?: A summary of alcohol treatment outcome research. In R. K. Hester & W. R. Miller (Eds.), *Handbook of alcoholism treatment approaches: Effective alternatives* (3rd ed., pp. 13–63). Allyn & Bacon.

Miller, W. R., Yahne, C. E., Moyers, T. B., Martinez, J., & Pirritano, M. (2004). A randomized trial of methods to help clinicians learn motivational interviewing. *Journal of Consulting and Clinical Psychology, 72*(6), 1050–1062.

Moore, M., Wolever, R., Hibbard, J., & Lawson, K. (2012). *Three pillars of health coaching: Patient activation, motivational interviewing and positive psychology.* Healthcare Intelligence Network.

Morton, K., Beauchamp, M., Prothero, A., Joyce, L., Saunders, L., Spencer-Bowdage, S., . . . Pedlar, C. (2015). The effectiveness of motivational interviewing for health behaviour change in primary care settings: A systematic review. *Health Psychology Review, 9*(2), 205–223.

Moyer, A., Finney, J. W., Swearingen, C. E., & Vergun, P. (2002). Brief interventions for alcohol problems: A meta-analytic review of controlled investigations in treatment-seeking and non-treatment-seeking populations. *Addiction, 97*(3), 279–292.

Moyers, T. B., & Martin, T. (2006). Therapist influence on client language during motivational interviewing sessions. *Journal of Substance Abuse Treatment, 30*(3), 245–252.

Mun, E.-Y., Atkins, D. C., & Walters, S. T. (2015). Is motivational interviewing effective at reducing alcohol misuse in young adults?: A critical review of Foxcroft et al. (2014). *Psychology of Addictive Behaviors, 29*(4), 836–846.

Naar-King, S., Parsons, J. T., & Johnson, A. M. (2012). Motivational interviewing targeting risk reduction for people with HIV: A systematic review. *Current HIV/AIDS Reports, 9*(4), 335–343.

Naar-King, S., & Suarez, M. (Eds.). (2011). *Motivational interviewing with adolescents and young adults.* Guilford Press.

Nuss, K., Moore, K., Nelson, T., & Li, K. (2021). Effects of motivational interviewing and wearable fitness trackers on motivation and physical activity: A systematic review. *American Journal of Health Promotion, 35*(2), 226–235.

O'Halloran, P. D., Blackstock, F., Shields, N., Holland, A., Iles, R., Kingsley, M., . . . Taylor, N. F. (2014). Motivational interviewing to increase physical activity in people with chronic health conditions: A systematic review and meta-analysis. *Clinical Rehabilitation, 28*(12), 1159–1171.

Olson, M. K. (2015). *Motivational interviewing in care and general health care settings: A meta-analysis.* Master's thesis, University of Wisconsin–Milwaukee. http://dc.uwm.edu/etd/827.

Pace, B. T., Dembe, A., Soma, C. S., Baldwin, S. A., Atkins, D. C., & Imel, Z. E. (2017). A multivariate meta-analysis of motivational interviewing process and outcome. *Psychology of Addictive Behaviors, 31*(5), 524–533.

Palacio, A., Garay, D., Langer, B., Taylor, J., Wood, B. A., & Tamkariz, L. (2016). Motivational interviewing improves medication adherence: A systematic review and meta-analysis. *Journal of General Internal Medicine, 31*(8), 929–940.

Phillips, A. S., & Guarnaccia, C. A. (2020). Self-determination theory and motivational interviewing interventions for type 2 diabetes prevention and treatment: A systematic review. *Journal of Health Psychology, 25*(1), 44–66.

Poudel, N., & Kavookjian, J. (2018). Motivational interviewing as a strategy for smoking cessation among adolescents—A systematic review. *Value in Health, 21*(Suppl. 1), S238–S239.

Poudel, N., Kavookjian, J., & Scalese, M. J. (2020). Motivational interviewing as a strategy to impact outcomes in heart failure patients: A systematic review. *Patient–Patient Centred Outcomes Research, 13*(1), 43–55.

Pourebrahim-Alamdari, P., Mehrabi, E., Nikkhesal, N., Nourizadeh, R., Esmaeilpour, K., & Mousavi, S. (2021). Effectiveness of motivationally tailored interventions on cervical cancer screening: A systematic review and meta-analysis. *International Journal of Women's Health and Reproduction Sciences, 9*(1).

Pudkasam, S., Feehan, J., Talevski, J., Vingrys, K., Polman, R., Chinlumprasert, N., . . . Apostolopoulos, V. (2021). Motivational strategies to improve adherence to physical activity in breast cancer survivors: A systematic review and meta-analysis. *Maturitas, 152*, 32–47.

Purath, J., Keck, A., & Fitzgerald, C. E. (2014). Motivational interviewing for older adults in primary care: A systematic review. *Geriatric Nursing, 35*(3), 219–224.

Rains, S. A. (2013). The nature of psychological reactance revisited: A meta-analytic review. *Human Communication Research, 39*(1), 47–73.

Rakel, D. (2018). *The compassionate connection: The healing power of empathy and mindful listening.* Norton.

Randall, C. L., & McNeil, D. W. (2017). Motivational interviewing as an adjunct to cognitive behavior therapy for anxiety disorders: A critical review of the literature. *Cognitive & Behavioral Practice, 24*(3), 296–311.

Ren, Y., Yang, H., Browning, C., Thomas, S., & Liu, M. (2014). Therapeutic effects of motivational interviewing on blood pressure control: A meta-analysis of randomized controlled trials. *International Journal of Cardiology, 172*(2), 509–511.

Resnicow, K., McMaster, F., & Rollnick, S. (2012). Action reflections: A client-centered technique to bridge the WHY-HOW transition in motivational interviewing. *Behavioural and Cognitive Psychotherapy, 40*(4), 474–480.

Resnicow, K., Sonneville, K. R., & Naar, S. (2018). The heterogeneity of MI interventions studies for treatment of obesity. *Pediatrics, 142*(5), e20182471.

Riper, H., Andersson, G., Hunter, S. B., de Wit, J., Berking, M., & Cuijpers, P. (2014). Treatment of comorbid alcohol use disorders and depression with cognitive-behavioural therapy and motivational interviewing: A meta-analysis. *Addiction, 109*(3), 394–406.

Rollnick, S., Heather, N., & Bell, A. (1992). Negotiating behavior change in medical settings: The development of brief motivational interviewing. *Journal of Mental Health, 1*(1), 25–37.

Romano, M., & Peters, L. (2015, June). Evaluating the mechanisms of change in motivational interviewing in the treatment of mental health problems: A review and meta-analysis. *Clinical Psychology Review, 38*, 1–12.

Rosengren, D. B. (2018). *Building motivational interviewing skills: A practitioner workbook* (2nd ed.). Guilford Press.

Rubak, S., Sandbaek, A., Lauritzen, T., & Christensen, B. (2005). Motivational interviewing: A systematic review and meta-analysis. *British Journal of General Practice, 55*(513), 305–312.

Saitz, R., Larson, M. J., LaBelle, C., Richardson, J., & Samet, J. H. (2008). The case for chronic disease management for addiction. *Journal of Addiction Medicine, 2*(2), 55–65.

Samson, J. E., & Tanner-Smith, E. E. (2015). Single-session alcohol interventions for heavy drinking college students: A systematic review and meta-analysis. *Journal of Studies on Alcohol and Drugs, 76*(4), 530–543.

Schaefer, M. R., & Kavookjian, J. (2017). The impact of motivational interviewing on adherence and symptom severity in adolescents and young adults with chronic illness: A systematic review. *Patient Education and Counseling, 100*(12), 2190–2199.

Schumacher, J. A., Williams, D. C., Burke, R. S., Epler, A. J., Simon, P., & Coffey, S. F. (2018). Competency-based supervision in motivational interviewing for advanced psychology trainees: Targeting an a priori benchmark. *Training and Education in Professional Psychology, 12*(3), 149–153.

Schwalbe, C. S., Oh, H. Y., & Zweben, A. (2014). Sustaining motivational interviewing: A meta-analysis of training studies. *Addiction, 109*(8), 1287–1294.

Shah, A., Jeffries, S. K., Cheatham, L. P., Hasenbein, W., Creel, M., Nelson-Gardell, S., & White-Chapman, N. (2018). Partnering with parents: Reviewing the evidence for motivational interviewing in child welfare. *Families in Society, 100*(4), 104438941880345.

Sherman, D. K., & Cohen, G. L. (2006). The psychology of self-defense: Self-affirmation theory. In M. P. Zanna (Ed.), *Advances in experimental social psychology* (Vol. 38, pp. 183–242). Academic Press.

Sinek, S. (2014). *Leaders eat last: Why some teams pull together and others don't*. Penguin.

Singh Ospina, N., Phillips, K. A., Rodriguez-Gutierrez, R., Castaneda-Guarderas, A., Gionfriddo, M. R., Branda, M. E., & Montori, V. M. (2019). Eliciting the patient's agenda—secondary analysis of recorded clinical encounters. *Journal of General Internal Medicine, 34*(1), 36–40.

Snape, L., & Atkinson, C. (2016). The evidence for student-focused motivational interviewing in educational settings: A review of the literature. *Advances in School Mental Health Promotion, 9*(2), 119–139.

Soderlund, L. L., Madson, M. B., Rubak, S., & Nilsen, P. (2011). A systematic review of motivational interviewing training for general health care practitioners. *Patient Education and Counseling, 84*(1), 16–26.

Sokalski, T., Hayden, K. A., Raffin Bouchal, S., Singh, P., & King-Shier, K. (2020). Motivational interviewing and self-care practices in adult patients with heart failure: A systematic review and narrative synthesis. *Journal of Cardiovascular Nursing, 35*(2), 107–115.

Song, D., Xu, T.-Z., & Sun, Q.-H. (2014). Effect of motivational interviewing on self-management in patients with type 2 diabetes mellitus: A meta-analysis. *International Journal of Nursing Sciences, 1*(3), 291–297.

Spencer, J. C., & Wheeler, S. B. (2016). A systematic review of motivational interviewing interventions in cancer patients and survivors. *Patient Education and Counseling, 99*(7), 1099–1105.

Spoelstra, S. L., Schueller, M., Hilton, M., & Ridenour, K. (2015). Interventions combining motivational interviewing and cognitive behaviour to promote-medication adherence: A literature review *Journal of Clinical Nursing, 24*(9–10), 1163–1173.

Stallings, D. T., & Schneider, J. K. (2018). Motivational interviewing and fat consumption in older adults: A meta-analysis. *Journal of Gerontological Nursing, 44*(11), 33–43.

Steinberg, M. P., & Miller, W. R. (2015). *Motivational interviewing in diabetes care.* Guilford Press.

Steinka-Fry, K. T., Tanner-Smith, E. E., & Hennessy, E. A. (2015). Effects of brief alcohol interventions on drinking and driving among youth: A systematic review and meta-analysis. *Journal of Addiction & Prevention, 3*(1).

Stott, N., Rollnick, S., Rees, M., & Pill, R. (1995). Innovation in clinical method: Diabetes care and negotiating skills. *Family Practice, 12*(4), 413–418.

Tanner-Smith, E. E., & Lipsey, M. W. (2015). Brief alcohol interventions for adolescents and young adults: A systematic review and meta-analysis. *Journal of Substance Abuse Treatment, 51*, 1–18.

Tanner-Smith, E. E., & Risser, M. D. (2016). A meta-analysis of brief alcohol interventions for adolescents and young adults: Variability in effects across alcohol measures. *American Journal of Drug and Alcohol Abuse, 42*(2), 140–151.

Tanner-Smith, E. E., Steinka-Fry, K. T., Hennessy, E. A., Lipsey, M. W., & Winters, K. C. (2015). Can brief alcohol interventions for youth also address concurrent illicit drug use?: Results from a meta-analysis. *Journal of Youth and Adolescence, 44*(5), 1011–1023.

Teeter, B. S., & Kavookjian, J. (2014). Telephone-based motivational interviewing for medication adherence: A systematic review. *Translational Behavioral Medicine, 4*(4), 372–381.

Thepwongsa, I., Muthukumar, R., & Kessomboon, P. (2017). Motivational interviewing by general practitioners for type 2 diabetes patients: A systematic review. *Family Practice, 34*(4), 376–383.

Thompson, D. R., Chair, S. Y., Chan, S. W., Astin, F., Davidson, P. M., & Ski, C. F. (2011). Motivational interviewing: A useful approach to improving cardiovascular health? *Journal of Clinical Nursing, 20*(9–10), 1236–1244.

Uzun, S., & Özmaya, E. (in press). The effect of motivational interview conducted by nurses on quality of life: Meta-analysis. *Perspectives in Psychiatric Care.*

Vallabhan, M. K., Jimenez, E. Y., & Kong, A. S. (2018). Motivational Interviewing for treating overweight and obese youth: A systematic review. *Journal of Adolescent Health, 62*(2, Suppl.), S119–S120.

Van Dorsten, B. (2007). The use of motivational interviewing in weight loss. *Current Diabetes Reports, 7*(5), 386–390.

VanBuskirk, K. A., & Wetherell, J. L. (2014). Motivational interviewing with primary care populations: A systematic review and meta-analysis. *Journal of Behavioral Medicine, 37*(4), 768–780.

Vasilaki, E. I., Hosier, S. G., & Cox, W. M. (2006). The efficacy of motivational interviewing as a brief intervention for excessive drinking: A meta-analytic review. *Alcohol & Alcoholism, 41*(3), 328–335.

Villarosa-Hurlocker, M. C., O'Sickey, A. J., Houck, J. M., & Moyers, T. B. (2019). Examining the influence of active ingredients of motivational interviewing on client change talk. *Journal of Substance Abuse Treatment, 96,* 39–45.

Wagner, C. C., & Ingersoll, K. S. (2013). *Motivational interviewing in groups.* Guilford Press.

Wagoner, S. T., & Kavookjian, J. (2017). The influence of motivational interviewing on patients with inflammatory bowel disease: A systematic review of the literature. *Journal of Clinical Medicine Research, 9*(8), 659–666.

Walthers, J., Janssen, T., Mastroleo, N. R., Hoadley, A., Barnett, N. P., Colby, S. M., & Magill, M. (2019). A sequential analysis of clinician skills and client change statements in a brief motivational intervention for young adult heavy drinking. *Behavior Therapy, 50*(4), 732–742.

Watkins, C. L., Wathan, J. V., Leathley, M. J., Auton, M. F., Deans, C. F., Dickinson, H. A., . . . Lightbody, C. E. (2011). The 12-month effects of early motivational interviewing after acute stroke: A randomized controlled trial. *Stroke, 42*(7), 1956–1961.

Wileman, V., Farrington, K., Chilcot, J., Norton, S., Wellsted, D. M., Almond, M. K., . . . Armitage, C. J. (2014). Evidence that self-affirmation improves phosphate control in hemodialysis patients: A pilot cluster randomized controlled trial. *Annals of Behavioral Medicine, 48*(2), 275–281.

Wilk, A. I., Jensen, N. W., & Havighurst, T. C. (1997). Meta-analysis of randomized control trials addressing brief interventions in heavy alcohol drinkers. *Journal of General Internal Medicine, 12*(5), 274–283.

Wilson, A., Nirantharakumar, K., Truchanowicz, E. G., Surenthirakumaran,

R., MacArthur, C., & Coomarasamy, A. (2015). Motivational interviews to improve contraceptive use in populations at high risk of unintended pregnancy: A systematic review and meta-analysis. *European Journal of Obstetrics, Gynecology, and Reproductive Biology, 191,* 72–79.

Winkley, K., Ismail, K., Landau, S., & Eisler, I. (2006). Psychological interventions to improve glycaemic control in patients with type 1 diabetes: Systematic review and meta-analysis of randomised controlled trials. *British Medical Journal, 333*(7558), 65.

Wong-Anuchit, C., Chantamit-o-pas, C., Schneider, J. K., & Mills, A. C. (2019). Motivational interviewing–based compliance/adherence therapy interventions to improve psychiatric symptoms of people with severe mental illness: Meta-analysis. *Journal of the American Psychiatric Nurses Association, 25*(2), 122–133.

Zomahoun, H. T., Guenette, L., Gregoire, J. P., Lauzier, S., Lawani, A. M., Ferdynus, C., . . . Moisan, J. (2016). Effectiveness of motivational interviewing interventions on medication adherence in adults with chronic diseases: A systematic review and meta-analysis. *International Journal of Epidemiology, 46*(2), 589–602.

Zulman, D. M., Haverfield, M. C., Shaw, J. G., Brown-Johnson, C. G., Schwartz, R., Tierney, A. A., . . . Verghese, A. (2020). Practices to foster physician presence and connection with patients in the clinical encounter. *Journal of the American Medical Association, 323*(1), 70–81.

Index

Note. Page numbers in *italics* indicate a figure or a table.

Lightning Source UK Ltd.
Milton Keynes UK
UKHW042006181122
412445UK00002B/17

9 781462 550388